GW00374283

LITTLE-KNOWN SECRETS OF HEALTH AND LONG LIFE

LITTLE-KNOWN SECRETS OF HEALTH AND LONG LIFE

BY STEVE PROHASKA

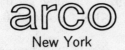
arco
New York

Published by Arco Publishing Company, Inc.
219 Park Avenue South, New York, N.Y. 10003

Copyright © 1972 by Stephen N. Prohaska

All rights reserved

Library of Congress Catalog Card Number 70-171671
ISBN 0-668-02530-1

Printed in the United States of America

introduction

This book has a most pleasant purpose—to show you and your family how to avoid doctors, dentists, hospitals, operations, and medical bills. In place of these burdens, this book offers you and your loved ones the opportunity to gain the greatest of all blessings: good health and long life. These glorious gifts are now attainable by those who desire them. Today, scientists are proving that your body can be made either more disease-prone or more disease-resistant. A multitude of exciting discoveries is already helping an enlightened few to achieve extraordinary health and longer life through simple, natural means.

I have been collecting these simple secrets of good health and long life through my thirty-eight years of study and research. Each time I discovered a new health and longevity secret, I was more elated than a prospector who discovers a nugget of pure gold.

All these wonderful secrets can now become yours. I'll tell you the things you do every day that undermine your health and shorten your life. I'll show you how to replace these harmful practices with simple measures that strengthen your health and prolong your life.

This book will show you how to make many wondrous changes within your body. These magical internal alterations will automatically bring you better health.

You've seen before-and-after pictures that show people who have successfully remodeled the appearance of their bodies—the fat lady who reduced her body to sylphlike proportions, the skinny weakling who built his body into a mass of muscle.

Such pictures illustrate *visible* bodily changes. This book will show you how to make *invisible* bodily changes. These alterations will be even more remarkable than those accomplished by the fat lady and the skinny weakling, even though you won't be able to prove your transformation with before-and-after pictures. On the other hand, you probably *will* be able to; people who become healthier, usually also become better looking. Nonetheless, the changes will be there inside you, where they count, bringing you better health and longer life.

In addition to these wonderful physical benefits, another kind of benefit can also be gained. This extra reward is something that accompanies superior health. It is a transformation in the way you *feel*. Improving the health somehow improves the spirits. Those who achieve better health can't help noticing a corresponding improvement in their mental outlook. Possessing this pleasant state of mind makes my way of living not only more healthful, but also more enjoyable.

But on top of this great feeling of well-being, there is something more—a great feeling of elation. This strange and wonderful phenomenon is known as "euphoria." Euphoria is the deeply satisfying feeling of exhilaration that goes beyond that of mere well-being. The sensation of euphoria has been variously described as a feeling of sheer bliss, exaltation and extraordinary well-being.

The feeling of euphoria is hard to put into words, but you'll recognize it when you experience it.

In addition to helping you improve your health and feel better, this book will show you how to enjoy these benefits *longer*.

It is no exaggeration to say that the information in these pages may bring you ten, twenty, thirty, or even more years of added life. Science has proved that certain harmful procedures can shorten life, while various beneficial actions can lengthen life.

For example, avoiding one common practice adds an average of eight years to human life, evading another pitfall adds a whopping nineteen years to the average person's lifetime, changing another practice adds an average of 17% to the person's life span, and another change adds five years to the average lifetime. These are facts backed by scientific research.

Many other practices can also contribute to longer life. Obviously, changing faulty living habits to beneficial ones may result in decades of extra life, and in some cases could actually double the lifetime.

The part you may find most difficult to accept about my system of health and longevity is its simplicity.

In these days, when so many people are ailing and dying prematurely despite all the wonders of medical science, you may find it hard to believe that you can achieve good health and longevity by means of your own simple efforts. Please don't be fooled because my program is plain and simple. Uncomplicated though it is, it works for others, and it can work for you.

The very simplicity of my living method can make your life not only more healthful but also *easier*. Your way of life is, quite likely, more difficult and more complicated than it need be. My simple way of living makes life easier, as well as more healthful and longer. It can make living more fun.

Contents

	Introduction	v
1.	The Enlightened Few	1
2.	Sick of Sickness	9
3.	The Odds Beaters	15
4.	Hang for Health	19
5.	The Broken Glasses	26
6.	The Insatiable Twenty Trillion	35
7.	The Biological Clock	42
8.	McCarrison's Comparisons	48
9.	Eat 'Em Alive	54
10.	The Staff of Death	63
11.	The Un-Food	72
12.	Have a Heart	79
13.	Fleshies and Veggies	84
14.	Unforbidden Fruit	91
15.	Milk and Egg Machines	97
16.	The Saturation Diet	103
17.	Too Few Chew	108
18.	The Mini-Menu	112
19.	The Pushers	115
20.	Invisible Invaders	120
21.	Avoiding the Assassins	130
22.	The Technocrats	142
23.	The Forgotten Art	147
24.	Health the Fast Way	151
25.	The Well Adjusted	156
26.	Help Yourself	162
27.	Take the Sting Out	171
28.	The Head in the Sand	176

29. The Drivers and the Conductors   180
30. Euphoria   188
31. Good Things Happen   194
32. Where, When, and How   201
33. Take It Off   211
34. The Bare-Skin Rug   216
35. The Health Belt   220
36. On Borrowed Time   224
37. The Ortho-Docs   226
38. The Malady Lingers On   230
39. The Mixed Bag   239
40. The Good Life   246
      Index   251

LITTLE-KNOWN SECRETS OF HEALTH AND LONG LIFE

one

The Enlightened Few

Many of the secrets of good health and long life have been open knowledge for years, but have been ignored by all but a wise few. Some of the secrets are generally recognized, but their full importance has been missed. Some were appreciated for a time, by a few at least, but lie now virtually forgotten.

Nevertheless, many good-health, long-life factors are being taken advantage of by a relatively small inner circle. Here and there, an enlightened few are practicing these secrets and attaining better health and extra years of life. The wise few depend on these obscure health secrets to defend themselves against heart trouble, to minimize the risk of cancer, and to bring them countless other health benefits. Many of those in the know even avoid colds and headaches. Let's take a look at some of the wise few who rely on simple measures to give them tip-top health and the ultimate in longevity.

1

H. L. Hunt is the richest man in America; many say the richest in the world. His fortune has been estimated at from between five hundred million and two billion dollars.

H. L. Hunt is also rich in another way—in health and longevity. Still in good shape at the age of eighty, Mr. Hunt is one of the informed minority who has long practiced some of the secrets advocated in this book.

Another insider who follows many of these health and longevity rules is Larry Lewis of San Francisco. Lewis is healthy enough to work as long as thirteen hours a day as a waiter; he precedes his working day with a six-mile run; yet he is one hundred and three years old!

Still another member of the enlightened minority, who has long followed most, if not all, of our secrets, is Paul Bragg of Burbank, California. When Bragg was but a teen-ager, his prospects of good health and longevity were almost nil. At age sixteen, doctors had given him up to die.

Instead, young Bragg discovered some of the secrets of health and longevity, applied them, and changed his life. He not only changed his life, he saved it. Instead of dying, he has lived on and on, year after year, in splendid health.

How old is Paul Bragg now? At this writing, he is eighty-nine, and he expects to live to be one hundred and twenty years old.

Is he still in good condition? He plays polo, swims a mile each day, runs two miles every morning, and does not even suffer from colds.

Harry Mason of Miami, Florida, is another man who had a poor chance of attaining longevity; nevertheless, he fooled the experts.

When Mason applied for life insurance at the age of twenty-one, he was turned down. But Mason stumbled onto some of the secrets of good health and long life. From then on, he practiced them faithfully.

How long has Mason lived—this man who was refused

life insurance at twenty-one? He recently celebrated his hundredth birthday.

My friend Phil Cohen became one of the enlightened few only after he was ready to cash in his chips.

At the age of sixty, Phil felt poorly, and his health was bad. Among the symptoms from which he suffered were chest pains, rectal bleeding, and varicose veins. Because he felt so distressed and suffered from so many alarming symptoms, he made out his will. Now ready to die, Phil Cohen prepared instead to live. He began practicing one of the secrets of health and longevity. "No doctor told me to do this," he says. "I just began doing it."

Immediately, Phil began to feel better. Soon, he was feeling excellent, free of his former symptoms. Vanished were the chest pains, gone was the rectal bleeding, smooth again were the once-varicose veins. Now, at age sixty-six, Phil is in such good condition that he can do many things he couldn't do when he was forty. One of these is playing three consecutive games of strenuous handball, another is swimming underwater for 120 feet.

Says Phil Cohen, "I'm a lot younger today at sixty-six than I was at sixty." And I agree. Though Phil has aged six calendar years, he has rejuvenated his body and subtracted far more than six years from his physical age.

These are only a few of the enlightened inner circle. Many other individuals have improved and prolonged their lives by adopting a good-health, long-life routine. You can do the same.

Sometimes entire families embrace a health and longevity plan, to the benefit of all. Let's discuss one family of eleven that takes advantage of our secrets.

The nine children in this family have had the advantage of being brought up on a good health program from birth. What have been the results?

A good check would be an examination of the children's teeth. Civilized mankind's most common ailment is dental decay. This disorder affects 98% of our country's population. Dental troubles frequently begin early in life. The average five-year-old has three decayed teeth; by age fifteen, he has eleven. In one survey of 2,536 children between the ages of one and twenty, only nineteen had perfect teeth—one out of one hundred and thirty-three. How does this compare with the dental record of the nine girls and boys in the health-minded family?

The odds against all these children having perfect teeth are astronomical. But this family has cheated the law of averages. Each of the nine children has grown up or is growing up without a cavity. Nine sets of perfect teeth. Not a cavity in nine mouths, not a penny for dental bills.

The case of the nine children with perfect teeth is quite familiar to me. I'm their father.

I haven't always managed to provide the Prohaska kids with all the material possessions they might have liked, but I have been able to give them something of far greater value: sound health and a good head start toward long life. So far, their physical troubles have been only occasional and minor. Recently, when one of the older children was filling out a questionnaire, she looked up in puzzlement and asked me, "Who is our family doctor?"

My system not only can *prevent* illness, as it has with my children, but it can also *cure*, as it did with the children's mother, Aline.

Before we were married, Aline suffered from chronic appendicitis. Her doctor advised an operation, which my wife-to-be kept postponing. After we married, under my influence, my new wife adopted some of my health secrets. The appendicitis attacks halted, never to return. The condition was cured simply and easily, without an operation.

Now, how has the head of the Prohaska family done on his health program?

A good basis of comparison is my condition today, at the age of fifty-six, to my state at age eighteen. At that age, I began, on a limited scale at first, my program of health betterment. Now that I am three times as old, I feel better than I did then.

Although I was in fair shape at eighteen, I suffered frequent headaches; they ended as soon as I adopted my new living habits. I was tired much of the time then; now I usually feel full of pep. I can hike 25 miles, run 13 miles, bicycle 60 miles.

Another health benefit I have managed to acquire purely by simple, natural means is to reduce substantially the rate of my heartbeat.

The rate at which the heart beats has been found to be associated with length of life. Dr. Raymond Pearl discovered, by checking the hearts of healthy, long-lived people, that one common trait was a relatively slow pulse.

Insurance company statisticians have learned that people with pulse rates of fifty-five to sixty-five live 20% longer than those with a rate of 70. Insurance companies seldom insure a prospect with a pulse rate higher than 100.

Why is a slow pulse associated with longer life? Because a slow pulse indicates that the heart is performing its work with less effort. The heart that beats slowly is strong and healthy and lasts longer.

The normal pulse rate, 72, can be materially reduced through practicing one of the secrets in these pages. Many people are able to lower their pulse rate to 60, 50, 40 or even fewer beats per minute. I have brought my own pulse rate down to 43.

I don't mean to imply that I expect to break any longevity records. Being a realist, I feel that my number may be up any day. However, long life is my goal.

Nor do I claim that my health is perfect. I get an occasional cold, and I have suffered many attacks of gout. Nevertheless, I am sure that my way of living has made me far healthier than I would be otherwise, and I am sure that this way of life has likewise benefited all my family.

The Prohaska family, in my thirty years of married life, has had little need for medical services. Not counting the costs of our numerous pregnancies and a few minor accidents, our total family medical expenses have come to only a few hundred dollars, but even this small sum might have been reduced through stricter health practices.

I've told you about our family's results, because I wanted you to witness the health benefits a family can attain. I want you to see that I am not just theorizing, but that I walk the same trail I recommend to others.

Now that we have visited a few of the enlightened minority, let's take a trip to an entire commonwealth of supremely healthy, long-lived citizens.

It is fortunate that our journey is on paper only, for the foreign state we will visit is almost inaccessible, being locked in by towering mountains. This state would be little noticed by the rest of the world were it not that its citizens are reputed to enjoy an existence almost free from sickness and to live almost invariably to extreme old age.

In northern India lies the tiny state of Hunza. Virtually all the 25,000 inhabitants of Hunza follow a health and longevity system almost exactly like the one I recommend. They do so not because someone has convinced them of the wisdom of this way, but because it happens to be their life style. Because the Hunzans are isolated from other people, they have developed their own way of living, uninfluenced by the practices of the rest of the world.

A few curious health-seekers from America and England have braved the arduous trip to Hunza to study its healthy inhabitants firsthand. They have returned with glowing accounts of the Hunzans' remarkable health and longevity.

A British medical researcher, Major-General Sir Robert

McCarrison, spent nine years observing the Hunzans and treating the few minor ailments they had. Dr. McCarrison reported: "I never saw a case of asthenic dyspepsia, of gastric or duodenal ulcer, of appendicitis, of mucous colitis, of cancer. . . ."

The healthy Hunzans form a striking contrast to ailing Americans. While the Hunzans have little or no need for medical services, in America sickness is an established part of our way of life.

According to *Time* magazine, ". . . . each year . . . 130 million Americans . . . pay 500 million visits to the doctor. For them, the doctors write a billion prescriptions for a total drug bill of some $3.5 billion. Each year, 27 million Americans go into a general hospital where they spend an average of 8.2 days and get a bill of $530, about half of which is covered by insurance. The total cost of U.S. medical care is now $53 billion a year—5.9% of the gross national product, or 7.5% of all personal income." [1]

Appalling as these figures are, they represent but a part of the total bill for disease in this country. *Time*'s figures cover only the direct costs of medical care. They do not take into account the resulting loss in wages and industrial production, nor the innumerable hidden costs, many of which it would be impossible to track down, let alone total.

But even the direct and indirect monetary expenses incurred as the result of illness do not represent the ultimate cost to our society. Though our physical troubles create a heavy drain on the nation's economic resources, the tremendous economic load is the least of the penalty. The cost in dollars can be reckoned, but the cost in human anguish is beyond computation. Who can place a dollars-and-cents value on human suffering?

If you are a typical disease-prone American, you can

[1] *Time*, February 21, 1969.

free yourself from many, if not most, of your physical problems. You needn't endure pain and suffering as a matter of necessity. You don't have to fritter away a sizable part of your income on medical care. You can become one of the enlightened few who keep medical services to a minimum, or even avoid them entirely.

SUMMARY

Your body can be made either more disease-prone or more disease-resistant through many simple factors. These simple secrets are helping an enlightened few to achieve good health and longevity.

two

Sick of Sickness

The recent past has seen a tremendous upsurge of interest in health. Today, one American in ten is health-minded. Millions of people are in search of better health, and they are trying to find it without consulting their physicians. Sales of exercise equipment have reached one hundred million dollars a year. Vitamin supplements are being sold in the amount of five hundred million dollars annually. A recently launched health magazine has had no trouble selling over a million copies per issue since the very first issue. These are signs that Americans are sick of sickness, that they are hunting for health. Since you are reading this book, you are also obviously one of the farsighted Americans who is seeking to better his health by forestalling sickness before it starts.

Because you are health-conscious and wish to learn the secrets of good health and long life, you could do what I did. For thirty-eight years, you could devote much of your spare time to study and research, and you could buy hundreds of books and thousands of periodicals and spend countless hours in libraries, including two of the country's

9

largest and most complete. You could pore through millions of words on health, longevity, and related subjects. Throughout those years, you could test your findings on yourself and on your family. You could do all those things, as I did.

Instead, you have chosen to read this book, which is *not* a medical book. Medicine is the study of disease, and I studied *health*, not disease.

The medical profession searches for the causes of disease; I searched for the causes of health. The medical profession doesn't study the healthy; it is kept too busy treating the unhealthy.

Much of what I have learned came from the study of information on the healthy and long-lived. What better approach to learning the secrets of a long, healthful life than to observe those who have achieved them? What, if anything, is different about their living habits? What discernible factors, if any, favor good health and long life? Are the healthful habits of these people, of the kind that can be copied to advantage by the rest of us?

Information on sickness is readily available, but literature concerning health and longevity is harder to find. Nevertheless, enough work has been done in this field to give us the answers we seek. The healthy and long-lived from many parts of the world have been sought out and interviewed. Their living habits have been checked and studied.

Some of the more outstanding investigations have been those which follow.

1. *Studies of United States residents over 95.* The 1950 United States census report showed about 29,000 persons over the age of 95. Of these, 402 were tracked down and quizzed by Dr. George Gallup, the well-known statistician, and his workers.

2. *Studies of United States residents over 100.* Of our country's 13,000 centenarians, 543 receive Social Security benefits. Most of the 543 have been interviewed by representatives from the Social Security Agency.

3. *Studies of residents of one area in Nebraska in which people live longer than anywhere else in the country.* Reporters from various periodicals have interviewed elderly residents of this area.

4. *Studies of Russian residents over 100.* The U.S.S.R. census for 1959 listed 21,708 people over one hundred years old. Information gathered from these oldsters is being studied extensively by the Russian government.

5. *Studies of the healthful, long-lived residents of Hunza.* The unusually long-lived Hunzans have been studied at firsthand by a number of doctors and scholars.

6. *Studies by Dr. Weston Price.* Dr. Price, a research dentist, investigated the living habits of healthy peoples in many parts of the world. Although his primary purpose was to find the causes of tooth decay, he found that good dental health was almost always accompanied by good general health.

7. *Studies by Dr. Raymond Pearl.* Dr. Pearl, of Johns Hopkins University in Baltimore, checked on the health practices of tens of thousands of long-lived people by means of personal examinations, questionnaires, and studies of death certificates.

In addition to the foregoing, a multitude of surveys have compared the healthy and the unhealthy and the long-lived and the short-lived in all walks of life. Moreover, countless scientific experiments have been done on animals which compare the effects of various factors on health and longevity.

The evidence emerging from this research is highly encouraging to the seeker of good health and long life. Yes,

the living habits of a majority of the old and healthy are
different from the average person's way of life in some re-
spects. Yes, certain factors (some of which, on the surface,
appear unimportant) often play a vital part in attaining
health and longevity. Yes, these favorable habits can
profitably be copied by those who aspire to good health
and long life.

My studies have led from researching the literature on
health to probing the living habits of the healthy and
long-lived and finally to investigating the basis for it all—
the evolution of man.

In the study of evolution can be found the reasons behind the secrets of good health and long life. The investigation of the living customs of the healthy and long-lived
teaches us *how*, the study of evolution teaches us *why*.
Only after we have traced back man's evolution can we
understand *why* modern man must follow certain eternal
laws if he is to enjoy a long and healthful life. The best
way to illustrate this is by the following example.

Nutritionists contend that good health and longevity
depend greatly on diet. To back up their claims, the nutrition-minded cite mankind's history. They point out that,
down through the centuries, man had subsisted on natural, unmodified foods: wild plants and wild game. Even
after man began to cultivate crops and domesticate animals, his food remained substantially unmodified. Simple
natural fare supported mankind for a hundred thousand
generations. Over the vast expanse of two million years
man's constitution adapted to and became dependent on
this type of diet.

However, recent generations have introduced radical
and extensive methods of altering food. Relatively over-
night, we began to change the composition of natural

foods. Through various refining and depleting processes, we now subject the structure of our foods to broad elementary changes. Man's constitution is powerless to adapt suddenly to these abrupt and sweeping dietary changes. Man has survived and thrived on natural foods for most of the time he has been on earth. His physical system still requires the unmodified foods on which the human race has survived for generations. The sudden switch to unnatural foods is the villain nutritionists blame for causing much unnecessary sickness and premature death. If your living habits are like those of most Americans, your quest for good health and long life is hindered by your refined and depleted diet.

However, nutrition is only one of many factors that influence your health and longevity. If you're a typical American, it is not only at meal time that you buck the forces of evolution. During most of your waking hours, and even while you sleep, you violate many laws of nature. Along with your depleted diet, you have adopted many other unnatural, harmful, and life-diminishing practices. These modern habits are poorly tolerated by a human constitution that was otherwise conditioned for over two million years.

Modern civilization brings us mixed blessings. With one hand, it brings us many benefits to health and longevity; with the other hand, it steals health and life from us. We must, while keeping civilization's many advantages, return, to some degree, to "uncivilized" living.

Beneath our thin veneer of civilization (the word itself goes back only about two hundred years), man is still basically the same animal he has been for two million years. His body can't and won't fully adjust to the many drastic innovations forced upon it by today's civilization. Instead of futilely trying to defy the unyielding forces of evolution, we must learn to live in harmony with natural, irrefutable laws. As the saying goes, "If you can't lick 'em, join 'em."

SUMMARY

Man's two-million-year evolution has established a living pattern which you must follow if you are to enjoy a long and healthful life.

three

The Odds Beaters

Let's consider, one by one, all the methods available to you for achieving better health and longer life.

One influence on your health and longevity differs from all the others, for it is the only factor you can't control by means of healthful living practices. This is your *heredity*. Someone has said that the best way to attain long life is to pick a pair of long-lived parents. This statement has a strong factual basis. That favorable heredity does contribute to longevity is indicated by studying the backgrounds of long-lived persons.

Dr. Pearl, Dr. Gallup, and others who have investigated the heredity of the healthy and long-lived, all came up with similar findings. The long-lived most often come from long-lived ancestors. In the Gallup study of the long-lived, for example, 26% had at least one parent who lived to be ninety or older, and, as might be expected, the family tree of the long-lived often included long-lived brothers, sisters, and grandparents. This is a strong indication of the importance of your heritage to length of life, for along with inheriting hair color or nose shape, we

15

apparently also may inherit the kind of constitution that
favors longer life. If you are the lucky offspring of long-
lived parents, you may have a head start toward your goal
of good health and long life.

But what if long life doesn't run in your family? Does
that mean one big strike against you?

No. A poor hereditary outlook is not necessarily a reason
for discouragement. Nearly one-fifth of those in the
Gallup study had no long-lived parent. Besides, even if
you come from a short-lived family, you can do a great
deal to counteract inherited defects. When I said that
your heredity was a factor you could do nothing about,
this was true only to a certain extent. In one sense, you
can do much about poor heredity. After all, your lineage
is only one of many factors influencing your health and
longevity. To overcome a poor hereditary background, you
will just have to try to exploit the other factors a little
harder. It may require extra effort, but the odds can be
beaten.

This is the story of one odd's beater.

Bernarr Macfadden, the famous physical culturist, has
inspiringly demonstrated that healthful living practices
can overcome poor heredity.

To find someone with a less favorable hereditary potential than Macfadden's would be difficult. His father died
when the boy was ten years old, his mother a few years
later. All of his brothers and sisters passed on when they
were middle-aged.

But Bernarr made himself the exception to the Macfadden rule. He followed a radically different kind of life
than that of his relatives. Far ahead of his time, he fer-
reted out many of the practices presented in this book.
Despite his family's tendency toward early demise, Macfadden lived to the age of eighty-seven. Had he had the

benefit of today's advanced longevity techniques, perhaps he might have lived even longer.

Some of those who enjoy a long, healthy life despite poor heredity apparently do so by sheer luck, but I think that investigation would show that such people usually happen to follow a living routine much like that recommended in this book. Simply through preference or circumstance, they practice many of the rules that contribute to good health and long life.

One such unwitting practitioner of the healthful way of life is Michael Sofka, a neighbor of mine, who is still healthy and active at ninety-one. Mike never suffers from headaches or stomach-aches. During each spring and summer, he spades, plants, and maintains just about the best backyard garden in the city. In the fall, he goes hunting. In the winter, he shovels his own sidewalk.

Last spring, after finishing his garden, Mike wanted more to do. So he came to the Prohaska yard and spaded and planted a garden for us. A short time later, when tree-cutters felled a large elm in the neighborhood, Sofka requested it for firewood. Using only handsaws, he cut up the tree into short lengths. These he split into thin pieces, using a wedge and a 15-pound sledge hammer. His mighty efforts produced a stack of firewood 6 feet high and 75 feet long. All this, mind you, at the age of ninety-one.

You can bet that I quizzed this young oldtimer about his ancestry and living habits. I learned that his parents had passed on so long ago that he doesn't remember how old they were when they died. He only remembers that he was eight when his mother died and sixteen when his father died.

Mike Sofka has attained longevity by means of his way

of life. Throughout his long life, he has practiced, for one reason or another, a style of living remarkably like the one about which you will read in the next chapter.

SUMMARY

The odds in favor of your living a long, healthy life are increased if your parents lived long. But even if you come from short-lived stock, the handicap can be overcome by practicing the good-health, long-life techniques that follow.

four

Hang for Health

Having discussed heredity, the one fixed factor, we can investigate those health and longevity influences that are subject to your control.

One good-health, long-life factor has to do with standing and sitting. Whether you stand or sit at your work may affect the length of your life. The study of work positions brings out a surprising and grim statistic. People who work in a standing position live shorter lives than those who work while seated. According to *Science News Letter*, those who work in a sitting position live an average of 17% longer than standees who perform the same work. This is a stiff price to pay for your work. It could mean dying in your middle eighties instead of living to be a hundred.

The reason why long hours of standing may shorten a person's life is not hard to guess. Standing for long periods hinders blood circulation. An upright position puts a strain on the heart and circulatory system, which must fight gravity in moving the blood from the lower extremities back to the heart.

To fix the blame for man's poorly engineered blood circulation requires a trip backward through time. Man evolved from a four-footed, apelike creature who lived in trees. During sixty million years of tree-living, apes moved about on four legs, feeding on a plentiful supply of fruit, leaves, and nuts, all of which were within easy reach.

When large-scale changes in weather conditions caused the forests to thin out, the ape was forced to move to the ground. There, he learned new feeding habits. Compelled to hunt food in order to survive, the ape-man assumed an upright posture, which freed his arms to carry and use weapons to hunt and for transporting food back to his mate and offspring. Gradually, over a period of uncountable generations, our ancestors, now more man than ape, became a biped.

Actually, the horizontal posture originated long before the ape even appeared on earth. Those who would disavow descent from the ape will probably derive scant consolation from the fact that, previous to our ape stage, we existed in an even lower form of life, for the ape evolved from a form of reptile that crawled on the ground. And even before our reptilian period, we swam in the seas as primitive forms of fish, only later to emerge on land. Evidence of man's beginning as a creature of the seas still exists today. At one stage, as the human embryo is forming, it temporarily possesses rudimentary gills.

As an upright citizen, you must contend with this precedent: The horizontal position goes back into time for incalculable eons, before the time of the ape, before the reptile stage, back to the very beginning of animal life in the seas.

Unfortunately, the ape-man from whom we descend adopted his erect posture only about two million years ago. In the opinion of many anatomists, this is not a sufficient period of time for man's system to have become fully adjusted to his present upright position.

What can you do to combat circulatory trouble, the enemy of the two-legged, short of learning to go around on all fours?

You can avoid long periods of standing. If your work requires long sessions on your feet, you would be wise to consider changing your vocation to one that allows you to sit at least part of the time. But if you can't or won't desert your standing job, perhaps your present work can be done while you are in a seated position. You may find it feasible to work while seated on a high stool that has high rungs on which to rest the feet. For example, housewives should work in a seated position whenever possible. Many household tasks, such as ironing and dishwashing, can be performed while sitting.

But even better for your circulation than sitting is work which involves moving about on your legs. Though standing, and even sitting for long periods, is a *hindrance* to circulation, moving about on the feet is an *aid* to circulation, for leg movement helps to move the blood.

Formerly, the work of moving the blood through the body was thought to be solely the work of the heart. Now it is known that bodily movements help circulate the blood. Contraction of muscles surrounding the veins in the legs produces a milking action, which helps to send blood back up to the heart. When you use your legs, you help your heart. The person who performs his work while on the move is healthier and lives longer than those who stand and even than those who sit. This has been proved in dozens of studies which compared the sedentary to the active.

When you must stand or sit for long periods, there is

a way to bring about the pumping action that helps keep the blood moving through the legs. Both standees and sittees can counteract gravity by flushing the leg veins every fifteen minutes or so, which can be done without pausing in the work.

First, rise up on your toes as high as possible, and then return to flat-footed position and raise the toes as high as you can. Repeat this several times. This exercise works all of the calf muscles, which helps to move the blood up toward the heart.

Another simple action will also combat gravity and clear the leg veins. Those who have the opportunity to interrupt their work now and then can reverse gravity's pull by taking a "gravity break." This heart-helping act need be performed only once each hour or two, perhaps during coffee breaks and at lunch time. Lie on your back and prop your feet up on something higher than your head—the higher, the better. Your leg veins will gain a respite in their battle with gravity, since gravity will be working in their favor for a change.

To combat still further the effects of gravity, some health-conscious stalwarts go beyond just raising their feet. They stand on their heads. Bernarr Macfadden, who lived to be eighty-seven, and George Bernard Shaw, who lived to be ninety-five, both made a practice of standing on their heads frequently. Paul Bragg, who is eighty-nine, has practiced daily headstands for many years, and he still does them for five minutes twice a day.

The easiest way to perform a headstand is with the help of a friend. After you have bent over and placed your hands and the top of your head on the floor in a triangular fashion, your helper raises your feet and holds them up for you. If you are agile, you may not need help. You may be able to achieve and hold this position by yourself, especially if you use a wall against your back for support. Watch out for back or neck damage. A cushion between your head and the floor will ease the strain on your head and neck.

In my personal war against gravity's damaging pull, I go even further than standing on my head. I use an advanced method that I feel sure brings even greater health benefits, even greater than raising the feet above the head, even greater than standing on the head. This is hanging upside down while suspended by the legs, a procedure which benefits not only the circulatory system, but also the spinal column. Man's spine, like his blood circulation, is a victim of his switch to an upright posture.

This change from horizontal to vertical has made the backbone vulnerable to the wear and tear of upright living. In its present position, the backbone supports the upper body, causing each bone to press on its neighbor below. Stresses and strains often cause these bones to move out of line, which results in pain and discomfort, and according to chiropractors, many other physical ailments that plague modern man.

Hanging upside down relieves the pressure of the spinal bones on one another. Instead of being forced together, the bones are stretched apart. The flattened cartilage between the bones is able to expand. The spinal column is stretched out more nearly to its true length. Spinal kinks hang out, like the wrinkles in a wash-and-wear shirt.

To hang yourself upside down, you will need to fasten a short length of metal bar or strong pipe in a horizontal position, at some distance above the floor. This bar will have to be at chest height, or higher. When you hang upside down, the bar is against the backs of the bent knees, for you hang suspended by the crooks of the knees.

When I first tried hanging upside down, the hard bar pressed so uncomfortably against the backs of my knees that I could hold the position only briefly. To make this process more agreeable, I wound soft padding around the bar and tied it in place.

One difficulty connected with hanging upside down is getting up into and down from the upside-down position. The trick is most easily accomplished with the aid of a rope fastened to the ceiling above the bar. This rope should touch the middle of the bar and reach a short distance below it. Knots in the rope make gripping easier.

To assume the upside-down position, the rope is gripped high up and the legs then raised into position. When the legs are in place, the hand grip is moved down along the rope until the body is lowered. Afterward, descent from the bar is accomplished by performing these actions in reverse. Both the bar and rope must, of course, be strong and securely fastened.

Hanging upside down produces a feeling of stimulation, as well it might, since it flushes the veins and stretches the spine. I find that it also brings quick relief from minor low-back pain.

The stunt is also said to be a good headache remedy. I wouldn't know, because I stopped getting headaches when I began my good-health program thirty-eight years ago. If you are a headache sufferer, it may be worth a try. Perhaps relief will be delivered through blood sent to the head by gravity.

Hanging upside down is the good-health, long-life secret that most fascinates the younger Prohaska children. Whenever I perform this feat, I can count on an amused but rapt audience.

If you decide to try hanging upside down, proceed with care. It is not an easy trick. Even if you are young and agile, you should try it only with caution. The inverted position should not be held for too long a period, perhaps only a few minutes—certainly not beyond comfort. If certain ailments are present, hanging upside down could be harmful instead of beneficial. If any doubt exists, consult your doctor before taking up the procedure.

If hanging upside down is too much for you, you can stretch your backbone in an easier way. The stretching is done in two installments. First, hanging by the hands from an overhead horizontal bar stretches the back from the shoulders down, and then, bending over from the waist while standing with knees bent stretches the upper spine and neck. The latter action also stimulates the blood circulation in the upper body and head.

Whichever method you adopt to fight the pull of gravity on your blood circulation and your spine, it need take only a few minutes a day.

SUMMARY

To combat upright posture's detrimental affects on health:

1. If possible, work in a seated position, or while moving about on your feet.

2. When standing or sitting for long periods, flush the leg veins by alternately raising heels and toes.

3. Every hour or two, pause briefly and prop the legs higher than the head.

4. To flush your circulatory system and, in the case of (b) and (c), stretch the spine: (a) perform headstands, (b) hang upside down, while suspended by the legs, or (c) alternately hang by the hands from a horizontal bar, and bend over from the waist while standing with knees bent.

five

The Broken Glasses

One source of health and longevity has been enjoyed by most preceding generations. Earlier man unknowingly absorbed health from overhead. Shining down on man for all of his two million years have been the healthful rays of the sun. Exposure to their influence through hundreds of thousands of successive generations has established in today's humans a need for sunshine.

Today, scientists are identifying the health-building forces in the rays of our sun. But despite our ever-widening knowledge of the sun's health benefits, we still spend most of our time indoors—at home, in school, wherever we work, in other public and private buildings, and in traveling between these places in cars. And even when we are outdoors, we usually cover ourselves with clothing, which keeps the sun's beneficial rays from reaching most of the skin. Ironically, the generation that knows the most about sunshine's health-giving qualities enjoys them the least.

One of the sun's health benefits is its tranquilizing effect on the nervous system, a force which can actually be felt. Relaxing in the sun brings a pleasant feeling of comfort. This sensation can be quite pronounced, and it has been noted by many. Science has certified that sunshine is a natural tranquilizer which has a calming, soothing effect on the nerves. Those who seek this effect from pills would do better to switch to sunshine.

Another of the sun's beneficial forces, identified years ago, is the action of the sun's rays on the human skin which produces within the body a substance vital to health and life. When activated by sunshine, the tiny blood capillaries lying near the skin's surface manufacture Vitamin D.

A shortage of Vitamin D can lead to a shortage of health. In a growing child, an extreme deficiency of Vitamin D may cause rickets, a bone disease that results in bowed or knock-kneed legs and a crooked spine.

Formerly only growing children were thought to be the only humans who required Vitamin D. Because the bones of adults had already formed, it was felt that they no longer were in need of this substance. Now, we know that the need for Vitamin D continues throughout life. Without enough Vitamin D, adults become vulnerable to osteomalacia, a softening of the bones, which is often called "adult rickets."

Vitamin D is available not only from the sun, but also from food. However, the only natural food which contains more than minute quantities of Vitamin D is fish-liver oil, so it would seem that for his Vitamin D requirements, man has long had to depend primarily on sunshine.

Nowadays, milk and several other commonly used foods are enriched with synthetic Vitamin D, so rickets has become rare. You probably get enough of this vitamin to escape rickets, which is caused by an *extreme* deficiency, but you may not be getting enough Vitamin D to prevent a *borderline* deficiency. Unless you secure an ample amount of Vitamin D, you may not get enough to protect your body against certain marginal ailments, such as tooth decay.

To be on the safe side, get plenty of sunshine. Don't depend on the Vitamin D you get from food sources and thus miss out on the possibly yet-undiscovered healthful effects of sunshine.

One hitherto unknown benefit from the sun's rays was discovered only a few years ago. Like many revolutionary discoveries, this one was an accident.

Dr. John Ott, who was severely crippled by arthritis, could walk only with the aid of a cane. Many arthritics have claimed to find relief in sunbathing, so Dr. Ott retired to Florida, where he hoped that exposure to strong sunshine might benefit his condition. However, although Dr. Ott sunned himself religiously, his ailment failed to improve. Then one day, he accidentally broke his sunglasses. Thereafter, his condition began to improve. By continuing to sunbathe without wearing glasses, Dr. Ott was soon able to throw away his cane. Apparently the sunglasses that had sheltered Dr. Ott's eyes from the sun's rays had also prevented something beneficial from entering his body. The sunglasses had blocked what must have been the only path available for this miraculous power. Thus, Dr. John Ott stumbled on an exciting new discovery.

It has long been known that ordinary glass blocks out the sun's beneficial ultraviolet rays. Now, it is also obvious that something in the sun's rays which is of benefit to bodily health can enter only through the eyes. This strange phenomenon is being investigated by Dr. Ott and others.

In discussing Dr. Ott's work, *Popular Science* magazine said: "A lack of natural light may be shortening the life of civilized man, impairing his health, reducing reproduction, and even inviting cancer."

Popular Science goes on to quote expert opinion to the effect that exposure to sunlight may increase one's life span: "Man developed in tropical areas of strong sunlight, and it could be that his life span is increased when he is exposed to reasonable amounts of natural light. In a paper published by the Building Research Institute, Dr. J. D. Hardy says the penalty for shutting out even a small degree of natural light may be acceleration of the aging process."[1]

It becomes increasingly evident that we spend too much of our lives inside clothing and behind windows, windshields, and spectacles. Sunshine allowed to shine on our skins and enter our eyes may well be helpful in alleviating or eradicating many of our illnesses.

But even better than alleviation or cure is the sun's power of *prevention*. Just a little sunshine prevents rickets. An *abundance* of the sun's rays may well help to prevent many other ailments.

As time goes on, scientists learn more and more about the sun's health-building qualities. But all of Old Sol's secrets may never be found out. In the meantime, nothing should stop you from frequently soaking up the sun's many health-building, life-saving benefits, both known and unknown.

No matter how busy you may be with indoor work, you can probably steal at least a short time in the sun, near the middle of the day when the rays are strongest. This

---

[1] *Popular Science*, February, 1969.

brief recess will give you some of the sun's health rewards, plus a few moments of relaxation. If you can spare more time, so much the better.

Lucky is the man with an outdoor job. On fair days, he automatically receives long exposure to the sun, just as early man did. The indoor worker must take advantage of his nonworking hours. The housewife's opportunities are better. She can arrange her daily schedule to allow her time in the sun. Children can also easily find time for fun in the sun. They would be better off if, instead of exposing themselves to the possibly harmful rays of television, they would bask in the beneficial rays of the sun.

When sunning yourself, you should make sure the healthful rays enter your eyes, and so you should not wear sunglasses. Face the sun at least part of the time, but don't stare directly at it, even if you can tolerate doing so. This is a dangerous action that can in time destroy your eyesight. You can get the sun's beneficial influence into your eyes simply by facing in the general direction of the sun.

To take full advantage of all the sun's good work, known and unknown, wear as little clothing as possible. Early man wore none at all.

In winter, sunning should be continued, even in cold climates. Although the body is clothed, Vitamin D benefits, and perhaps yet-unknown benefits, still enter the body through the portions of it that are exposed, such as your cheeks. It is in the cheeks that the capillaries lie closest to the surface, which gives sunshine the best opportunity to create Vitamin D.

To explain the thinness of the skin on human cheeks, I advance the following theory. Thin cheek skin is apparently an evolutionary development created by the body's need for Vitamin D. In the days when people went unclothed, they exposed all of the skin's surface to the sun, but when they began to wear clothing, they blocked the sunshine from much of their bodies. Some of the skin was perhaps already hidden by long hair, and in the case of adult males, by whiskers. But this still left the cheeks exposed. Those who happened to have the thinnest cheek skin received the most Vitamin D. They were the ones most likely to survive to reproductive age. Their children inherited the tendency to thin cheek skin; thus, the attribute was not only passed along, but enhanced.

Take advantage of your thin cheek skin, and get out in the sun even in winter.

Since I have recommended sun worship, I must warn you against *too much* of a good thing and caution you against overexposure. While frequent exposure to the sun's rays is beneficial, prolonged sunning can be harmful, and it must be avoided.

You have perhaps experienced one of the unpleasant results of prolonged exposure: sunburn. To guard against sunburn, exposure should begin with only ten minutes or so the first day. On succeeding days, the time can be gradually lengthened. Frequent change of position will lessen the risk of overexposing any one area of your body.

For maximum benefits from Vitamin D, sunbathing sessions needn't be lengthy. Too much of the direct sun may give you an overdose of Vitamin D, particularly in these days of Vitamin D food enrichment. Excessive Vitamin D intake causes your body to over-react, and too much sun may be harmful. A light or medium tan is a better indicator of correct Vitamin D dosage than a deep tan.

Prolonged sunbathing is particularly unwise during extremely hot weather. Enervation or, in extreme cases, heat stroke can be brought on by too much exposure to intense heat. The heat of the sun is no exception.

The skin of a baby is more delicate than that of an adult, and it is more sensitive to sunlight. Sunbaths for babies and young children should be of short duration. The top of a baby's head is especially sensitive to direct sunlight, and it should always be covered.

Overexposure, when continued over a long period of time, has been known to cause skin cancer. Doctors have had no difficulty in connecting skin cancer with over-exposure to the sun. Ninety percent of such cases occur on the face, neck, and other most-exposed areas, and skin cancer is five times as common in the southern states as in the rest of the country.

But skin cancer develops, if at all, only after years of excessive exposure. It need not be feared by the sensible sunbather.

All the preceding warnings apply to overexposure in *direct* sunshine. *Indirect* sunshine seems to provide much the same benefits as the direct sun—without the risks. Indirect sunshine is plentiful even in the shade. Sunlight is scattered in all directions by our earth's atmosphere. These scattered rays reach around corners and poke into shadows. In addition to this "sky shine," there are other sources of indirect sunshine, such as the reflective surfaces like sand and snow.

To gain the sun's health rewards in full measure, do as early man must have done: Spend some of your outdoor hours in the direct sun, the rest sunning in the shade.

Though the glass in windows blocks out virtually all the sun's beneficial ultraviolet rays, there are ways to bring these rays inside.

In summer, screened open windows permit the passage of some direct sunshine into your home. In winter, some of the sun's health advantages can also be enjoyed in the shelter of your home, perhaps even in your office or wherever it is that you work. One way is to open a window and sit near it. You'll lose some of the heat, but you'll gain a little healthful sunshine.

Another way to sun yourself indoors is by replacing window glass with plastic. This material allows penetration of most of the sun's beneficial ultraviolet rays. The windows most exposed to the sun are those which face south.

Replacing window glass with plastic need not be expensive. The thin, flexible material commonly sold for storm-window use will serve the purpose. Just remove the entire window, and tape the plastic over the opening. Even a single thickness admits more heat than it lets out, whenever the sun shines through it. The rest of the time, loss of heat can be diminished by taping a second layer of plastic to the window casing.

We Prohaskas soak up sunshine all year long through the south wall of our home. This wall is almost entirely of clear $\frac{1}{4}''$ plastic. Our kitchen, living room, and bedrooms all border on this wall. I purposely designed the building this way for two good reasons. The first reason was to expose us to the sun's benefits more often. The second reason for our plastic south wall is one of economy. This style of construction provides what is known as a solar house. A solar house is heated free of charge by the sun whenever it shines, even in midwinter. This is a desirable feature in upstate New York, where winter temperatures are often severe. Even on below-zero days, our heat is turned off whenever the sun is out.

Free solar heat is most often available on cold days, for it is usually on the coldest days that the sun is out, as you may have noticed.

"What about summer?" you may ask. "Doesn't the sun's heat become unbearable?"

No, because an automatic adjustment takes place. In

winter, the sun is relatively low, even at midday, and the rays reach far into the house. But in summer when the rays are more powerful, the sun's position is higher, and then its rays barely reach inside.

Nevertheless, living in a plastic-windowed solar house is no excuse for missing out on natural sunlight that is filtered only by air. Plastic may possibly screen out some still-to-be-discovered health elements, so if you build a solar house, admire it frequently from outside.

SUMMARY

The health benefits of sunshine enter the body by way of the skin and the eyes.

The rays of the sun shining on the skin produce at least two beneficial effects: Tranquilization of the nervous system, and production of Vitamin D, a substance necessary for health.

The rays of the sun entering the eyes produce health benefits not yet fully understood but now under scientific investigation.

In order to enjoy the sun's health benefits to the utmost: Sunbathe outdoors frequently all year long, spend part of the time in direct sunshine and part of the time in the shade, wear as little clothing as possible, don't wear glasses outdoors, don't overexpose yourself in direct sunshine, and let the sun into your home by opening windows or replacing glass with plastic.

six

The Insatiable
Twenty Trillion

Although you are seldom conscious that the process is
going on, you take air into your lungs about eighteen
times a minute, every minute of your life. If your lungs
suddenly became immobile, you would become aware of
discomfort within seconds, and in a minute or so, you
would be acutely uncomfortable. In three minutes, your
brain cells would begin to die, and in six minutes or less
you would be dead.

With every breath, you take into your lungs oxygen,
the gaseous substance on which your life depends. Your
bloodstream rushes this oxygen to every part of your body,
where it is eagerly gobbled up by each of your twenty
trillion cells. They depend on a constant supply of this
precious stuff for their survival and yours. Your body has
no way to store oxygen, so this vital element must be
taken in breath by breath constantly, day and night, as
long as you are to live.

But this is only half the story. While your blood is rushing oxygen from your lungs to each of your cells, it is also performing a second task imperative to your existence. As your cells consume oxygen, waste is produced. If allowed to remain, this refuse would soon choke to death both you and your cells. So your bloodstream's second job is to return the waste matter, carbon dioxide, to the lungs, where it is expelled. Thus, your bloodstream doubles as delivery boy and garbage collector.

As a result, there you are, breathing in and out twenty-two thousand times every twenty-four hours, feeding oxygen to trillions of insatiable cells and relieving them of the carbon dioxide they so desperately need to eject.

This process of breathing is performed more efficiently out-of-doors than indoors.

Fresh outdoor air consists of 20.9% oxygen and only .03% carbon dioxide. (The rest is nitrogen and argon.) Indoors, these percentages change. As people breathe, they use up oxygen. At the same time, they add carbon dioxide to the air. How much the proportions change depends on the size of the closed area and the number of people who are in it.

When the carbon dioxide content of indoor air is allowed to reach a concentration of 5% or so, which it sometimes does, it produces discomfort. At 10%, the discomfort becomes acute, and it can be tolerated for only a few minutes. At 25%, death results.

That death can occur from an oxygen-carbon dioxide imbalance was proved, as far back as 1756, by the well-known tragedy of the Black Hole of Calcutta. More recently, it has been proved by those unfortunate individuals who died as the result of being locked in airtight trunks of cars. One cool fellow in this fix saved his life by slowly letting air out of the spare tire.

Because severe air imbalance quickly results in the death of human life, it would seem to follow that even a minor imbalance might cause some harm, particularly if long-continued.

Indeed, this theory was proved years ago, though in reverse, by Dr. Millet, the Brockton, Massachusetts, physician who first demonstrated the value of fresh air as an aid to curing the tubercular. Dr. Millet prescribed a radical new treatment: sleeping outdoors. After a few months, despite the fact that Millet's outdoor-sleeping patients continued to work long hours indoors during the day, they improved greatly. The new therapy became widely adopted in the treatment of tuberculosis, even in cold climates. Many sufferers who lived outdoors day and night all year long recovered.

Perhaps indoor air won't cause you to contract tuberculosis, but it may do other dirty work inside your body. You may be in the same boat as the sun-starved person who gets enough Vitamin D to prevent rickets, but not enough to prevent other sickness, and perhaps premature death.

Oxygen-depleted indoor air may even be a contributor to the development of cancer. Consider the following evidence.

Many researchers believe that the basic cause of cancer is an inadequate supply of oxygen to the cells. One expert who holds this opinion is Nobel Prize Winner, Dr. Otto Warburg, director of the Max Planck Institute for Cell Physiology, Berlin-Dahlem, Germany. In 1955, Dr. Warburg stated in one of his lectures that a lifetime of research had convinced him that cancer was caused by depriving the cells of oxygen.

Dr. H. A. Schweigart, another German researcher, found that cancerous tissue always shows a deficiency of oxygen.

Inspired by the theory that oxygen deprivation may be

the direct cause of cancer, medical science is trying a
new method of treatment. Patients are placed in a pressure chamber where cancerous tissues are drenched with
oxygen. If this procedure proves effective, it would be
logical to suggest its use not only in treatment, but also in
the prevention of cancer. A daily stint of oxygen-drench-
ing might prevent cancer from developing. Those who
could afford the process might be kept immune from cancer.

To others, a free method of furthering oxygen intake is
available: the breathing of oxygen-filled outdoor air. By
giving the lungs more oxygen for delivery to the cells, a
plentiful consumption of outdoor air could conceivably
act as a deterrent to cancer. This is only a theory, but one
which deserves investigation.

As is the case with sunshine, oxygen-rich outdoor air
almost surely provides health benefits yet to be discovered. But you don't have to wait for their discovery.
You can get all of the outdoor-air's health rewards, known
and unknown, right now.

Early man spent all of his days and nights outdoors.
From him, you inherited a body that flourishes on outdoor
air.

Obviously, those who will gain the most health benefits
from outdoor air are those who spend most of their hours
out-of-doors. Unfortunately, this is an impossibility for
most people. Therefore, we must arrange our lives so as to
spend as much time as possible out-of-doors, breathing
the high-oxygen formula on which the human race grew
up.

During the hours that you must spend indoors, you can
minimize the effects of reduced oxygen supply by ventilation. Opening the tops or the bottoms of windows isn't
enough. The best circulation occurs when both the tops

and bottoms are open. Air change will be speeded by placing a fan near the top of a window, which will blow stale
air out at the top and cause fresh air to enter at the
bottom.

Even in cold weather, ventilation should not be neglected. For a change of air, throw your windows open
wide for a few minutes every hour or so. The room will
quickly regain its former warmth afterward.

At work, your boss or your fellow employees may not
appreciate fresh winter air. If you are stuck with impure
air during much of the day, you may still see that you have
lots of fresh air during the night hours. Protected from
the cold if necessary by heavy pajamas and plenty of
blankets, you can sleep with your windows open wide all
night long. The air you breathe, though not as beneficial
as pure outdoor air, will be better for your health than ordinary indoor air.

In addition to ventilation, there is another way to improve indoor air balance.

Outdoor air undergoes a constant process of purification. Trees, shrubs, and other plants breathe, but by means
of a process that is the opposite of man's. Plants *take in*
carbon dioxide and *expel* oxygen. Both house plants and
outdoor plants use this reverse breathing process, and adding house plants to your home can bring about a better
balance of air indoors. If you like plants, decorate your
home with them, and enjoy their health benefits along
with their beauty.

Even better than sleeping with windows thrown wide
open is sleeping on an open porch outdoors or in your
backyard. There, you can enjoy fresh outdoor air in all its
purity. All you need is a sleeping bag of the kind sold in
sporting goods stores. Sleeping bags are used by campers,
and they make a tent unnecessary. Heavily insulated bags

are available for outdoor sleeping during cold weather. With a sleeping bag, you can take a vacation from indoor air every night.

In fact, entire families would do well to become backyard habitués. Out in the yard, only seconds and steps away, await the health benefits of fresh air and sunshine. To gain more of the great health rewards of outdoor living, known and unknown, I recommend to your family the establishment of a backyard health center.

Constructing a patio or porch, which is at least partly roofed over, is not beyond the abilities of the average do-it-yourselfer. A large picnic table will provide a place for outdoor meals and other outside activities. A pool and toys, such as swings, a teeter-totter, or a slide, will encourage healthful outdoor living. Both your television and radio can be brought outside, as can reading matter and games.

Some work habitually performed indoors can be done just as well outside. Many household tasks, such as washing and ironing, can be done in the backyard or on a porch. (In the southern states, many housewives keep their washing machines on a patio in the backyard.) Schoolwork can be done on a picnic table. At night, fresh air benefits can be continued by making use of sleeping bags. While working, playing, and resting, you and your family can be gaining the health rewards of the great outdoors.

Backyard living can save more work than it creates. Wearing but little clothing saves on washing and ironing. Cookouts, with paper cups and plates, lessen dishwashing. Use of sleeping bags eliminates the chores of bedmaking. Informal backyard living is not only more healthful, but also pleasanter and easier.

That outdoor living encourages health and longevity seems to be indicated by observation of the healthy and long-lived. The majority of such people work or have worked at farming, which of course provides plentiful exposure to the benefits of sunshine and fresh air.

Many of the old-timers investigated by Dr. Gallup and by the Social Security Service had spent most of their years on farms. A preponderance of the Soviet centenarians lived in the province of Georgia, which is primarily agricultural. The Hunzans also live by farming. Moreover, the various primitives studied by Dr. Price were mostly farmers, hunters, or fishermen.

Like all of these healthy, long-lived people, you too can gain the benefits of sunshine and outdoor air. Both are free.

SUMMARY

In order to survive, you must constantly breathe in the fuel, oxygen, and expel the waste product, carbon dioxide. Outdoor air is rich in oxygen and low in carbon dioxide. Indoor air is lower in oxygen and higher in carbon dioxide.

To gain the health benefits of outdoor air, arrange your days so you can spend as much time outdoors as possible; when indoors, ventilate by opening windows; improve indoor air balance with house plants, and sleep at night with windows open or, better still, sleep outdoors in a sleeping bag.

seven

The Biological Clock

From early childhood, we are taught that the human body requires at least eight hours' sleep each night. Do the healthy old-timers surveyed follow this time-honored rule?

The majority do. Eighty-five percent of the senior citizens surveyed by Gallup habitually slept at least eight hours a night. Of these, 16% slept even longer—nine or ten hours each night. The Hunzans, we are told by those who have observed them, also average at least eight hours' sleep nightly.

A survey of healthy long-lived men and women made by the Life Extension Institute of Rutgers University produced a similar report. Regardless of their other living habits, most of the healthy oldsters got at least eight hours' sleep each night.

Further evidence that at least eight hours' sleep is required nightly comes from several surveys of normal sleeping habits. These investigations showed that, when allowed to sleep as long as they wish, most subjects sleep about eight hours.

Even in the Arctic regions, where the days are nearly twenty-four hours long during the summer, sleeping hours average nearly eight each day. Nathaniel Kleitman, a physiologist who specializes in the study of sleep, interviewed residents of northern Norway. He found that during the long-day season, they slept about seven hours a day. During the winter, when it is the *nights* that last nearly twenty-four hours, they slept about eight hours per night.

Another tally of sleeping hours involved twenty-five members of a British expedition based near the North Pole. During the twenty-four-hour nights, the explorers were allowed to sleep whenever they wished. After one month, the nightly average per man totaled 7.9 sleeping hours.

From all this, it would appear that the traditional eight hours' sleep is about the minimum adult requirement. Babies and growing children need still more, as proven by observation of their normal sleep habits.

But many of us, children and adults alike, not only don't get enough sleep, we *make sure* we don't. We manage this with the help of a fiendish device designed to prevent a normal full-night's sleep. One of the many diabolical inventions with which man steals from himself is the alarm clock. Without it, most people would probably find themselves sleeping about eight hours or more each night. With it, they rob themselves of health-building, life-lengthening sleep.

If your schedule doesn't allow time for a full night's sleep, I say that there is something wrong with your schedule. If you have allowed yourself to get caught up in a rat race of activity, I suggest that it is time for you to slow your life down to a more leisurely rate. Your frenzied pace is probably causing nervousness and tension, which, as will be demonstrated later, promote sickness and shorten life. A slower tempo will bring the necessary tranquility to your life and give you enough time for all the sleep you need.

Whatever has been keeping you up late often can just as well be done earlier. Even if it can't be, you may discover that whatever you used to stay up for is not missed much, especially when you get hooked on the habit of regularly enjoying a good night's rest. Instead of having your sleep cut unpleasantly short, you will get a full quota of health-building slumber. Instead of being prematurely jolted from sleep, you will waken naturally, refreshed and revitalized by that great tranquilizer, sleep.

If you must use an alarm clock, set it not to insure undersleeping, but to prevent oversleeping. In that way, your family can get all the sleep they need and still have time to make the commuter train and school bus.

Those who find themselves with a little extra time on their hands can step outside and enjoy a bit of the morning sunshine and fresh air.

To augment your nightly sleeping hours, I recommend that you also take a nap during the day whenever possible. I can't back up this advice with much evidence of its healthfulness. Although I have uncovered plenty of literature on sleep, little of it has dealt with nap-taking. I found a record of but one study that linked nap-taking with health. This survey indicated that the health of elderly people improved when they began taking naps. This is the only conclusive evidence I could find on the subject, but a dearth of information on nap-taking doesn't stop me from boosting it as a health improver. From my own experience, I know that a nap in the middle of the day brings renewed energy. I feel sure that this feeling of refreshment also demonstrates that naps help build health. Others share my belief, including the many doctors who recommend nap-taking to their patients.

Earlier, man slept on a firm, level surface, the ground. Modern man substitutes a soft mattress which rests on springs that often sag in the middle.

Some health-seekers have tried a firmer sleeping surface, more like that on which man slept for two million years, and found they slept better. Bernarr Macfadden slept on the floor for about seventy of his eighty-seven years.

You probably won't want to copy Macfadden's rigorous regimen, but you might want to do what many health enthusiasts have done. Replace your resilient bed springs with 3/4" plywood. Your lumber dealer will cut you some in the size needed to fit your bed. Next, replace your big, fat mattress with a thinner one. Now you can sleep on a padded, yet firm, surface more like the one on which 99% of your ancestors slept. (You can get the same effect with a sleeping bag laid on the ground or other firm, hard surface.)

Investigating the habits of the healthy and long-lived reveals not only the need for eight hours' sleep nightly, but also brings to light a curious fact about their sleeping customs. The healthy and long-lived go to bed early.

Almost 90% of those Gallup studied have habitually retired early and risen early. Most followed the custom of retiring by nine-thirty. The Hunzans follow a similar early-to-bed schedule. Their bedtime is listed by one investigator at seven or eight o'clock, and in the winter even earlier. The Hunzans' reason for going to bed early is a practical one. They have no electricity—or even kerosene or candles.

Primitive men must also have been early retirers. Like today's Hunzans, they had no lights. For two million years, people bedded down at the arrival of darkness or soon after. Their alarm clock was dawn. Without practical sources of artificial light, all but a relative few of even our most recent ancestors were, of necessity, early retirers and early risers. The Gallup oldsters' early retiring habits are perhaps a carry-over from their younger days when electric lights were unknown.

It may be hard to see the relationship between your health and longevity and the early-to-bed habits of generations long gone. Nevertheless, there appears to be a connection.

When you go to bed late, you may affect some sort of long-established inner biological rhythms which govern your body's functions. These rhythms may have long ago become an unalterable part of you, a part unaffected by a generation or two of late-retirers.

Dr. Rene Dubos, head of the Department of Environmental Biomedicine at New York's Rockefeller University, has observed these long-established biological patterns. In a *Reader's Digest* article condensed from *Life*, Dr. Dubos states: "Some of man's deepest biological traits are governed by the movement of the earth around the sun and of the moon around the earth, and by the rotation of the earth on its axis. We evolved under the influence of cosmic forces that have not changed." [1]

That an inner biological clock exists, and that its works can be disrupted, has long been observed by travelers in jet planes. After a long flight, passengers and crew often experience symptoms of mental inefficiency and physical distress. Rarely do the symptoms develop after moving

[1] *Reader's Digest*, October, 1970 (Condensed from *Life*, July 24, 1970).

north or south. They almost always occur after traveling east or west. Experts believe that the rapid movement (up to six hundred miles per hour) into earlier or later time zones is responsible for upsetting the body's natural biological rhythms.

Perhaps something similar happens to your biological clock when you go to bed late. Possibly whatever happens not only affects energy and efficiency, but health and longevity as well.

"Every hour of sleep before midnight is worth two hours after midnight," goes an old saying. And, as with many another old saying, there may be something to it.

SUMMARY

Encourage better health and longer life with these sleeping habits: Retire early in the evening, sleep at least eight hours each night, take a midday nap when possible, replace your bedsprings with plywood, and replace a thick mattress with a thinner one.

eight

McCarrison's Comparisons

We come now to the good-health, long-life factor that is almost unanimously considered most important by writers on health topics: nutrition.

It is one's diet, contend the nutritionists, that has more influence than anything else on health and longevity. Their theory is that man is what he eats, and if he habitually consumes those foods rich in the nutrients required by the human body, he will enjoy a long disease-free life. The unbiased can only agree that there is much logic in the argument that diet can greatly influence health and longevity. Moreover, the proponents of the nutrition theory have piled up mountains of impressive evidence to back their contentions.

I don't go all the way with the nutritionists, however, because I consider two other influences even more essential. But I will agree that of the factors we have discussed thus far, nutrition is, with the possible exception of heredity, by far the most important.

After asserting the advantages of good nutrition, many nutritional experts proceed to criticize the diet of most Americans. Its various shortcomings are responsible, they assert, for most of the physical troubles that beset us today.

But representatives of our food industry proclaim the present-day American diet the best the world has ever seen. These food distributors point out that modern food preservation methods and rapid transportation furnish fresh meats, fish, fruits, vegetables, and dairy products to all parts of the country the year round. The nutrition-minded agree that our excellent food preservation and distribution systems keep our stomachs full, but they add that a full stomach does not necessarily mean proper nutrition.

The unfortunate truth is that much of the food we eat is not very nutritional. It has suffered alteration that depletes it of vital elements. In many of the foods we eat today, the substances our bodies need for good health and long life are often in short supply, and are sometimes completely missing.

Robbing our food of nutrients is perpetrated in two ways: cooking and artificial refining.

The custom of cooking food came rather late in man's evolution. Commercial food refining and processing became common only during the past few generations.

The practices of cooking and refining damage or entirely remove many of food's natural nutrients. Yet it is on these now-reduced or missing nutrients that man's physical system evolved over a period of several million years, and it is on these now-reduced or missing nutrients that man's health and life substantially depend. The twin evils of cooking and refining are blamed by some doctors and nutritionists for many of modern man's ailments, from colds to cancer.

The isolated Hunzans, whose eating habits are virtually

unaffected by the outside world, have made excellent subjects for comparison of the health effects of raw, natural foods versus cooked, processed foods.

Because wood and other fuels are very scarce in their land, the Hunzans eat raw any food that can be enjoyed uncooked. Food refining, of course, is unheard of in the land of the Hunzans.

Probably the most thorough investigator of the Hunzans' living habits was Sir Robert McCarrison, a prominent English doctor who had been appointed Director of Nutrition Research in India.

For nine years, Dr. McCarrison lived and practiced among the Hunzans. In contrast to the residents of his native England, McCarrison found that the Hunzans "enjoyed a remarkable freedom from disease." What few ailments he was called upon to treat were mostly of a minor nature, or were injuries due to accidents. In the nine years he spent observing the twenty-five thousand or so Hunzans, Dr. McCarrison never saw even a single case of some of our common diseases.

To what did Dr. McCarrison attribute the Hunzans' remarkable freedom from disease? He gave credit to their natural diet. Even before studying the Hunzans, McCarrison had observed other healthy primitives and had come to the conclusion that the difference between good health and poor health was determined by food habits.

To prove his convictions conclusively, Dr. McCarrison set out to demonstrate them in his laboratory. His method was to feed one group of rats on a diet similar to that of the healthy Hunzans, while another group was given a faulty diet, similar to that commonly eaten in neighboring India.

McCarrison fed 1,189 rats on foods like those eaten by the Hunzans. The animals were given unrefined wholegrain bread, fresh raw vegetables, raw (unpasteurized) milk, and a little meat, together with the bones. At the same time, McCarrison fed 2,243 rats on a diet like that customarily eaten by the poorer classes of India.

How did each group of rats make out?

Those on a diet of unrefined and uncooked foods did marvelously. Here is part of Dr. McCarrison's report, as delivered to the Royal College of Surgeons in 1931.

"During the past two and a quarter years there has been no case of illness in this universe of albino rats, no death from natural causes in the adult stock, and, but for a few accidental deaths, no infantile mortality. Both clinically and at postmortem examination this stock has been shown to be remarkably free from disease. It may be that some of them have cryptic disease of one kind or another, but if so, I have failed to find either clinical or macroscopical evidence of it." [1]

Now, how did the *faultily-fed* rats fare?

Collectively, they developed just about every disease known. McCarrison made a list for the College of Surgeons, which mentioned sixty-one separate ailments and included diseases of every organ.

Since McCarrison's studies in the 1920's, his results have been verified by many other scientists. Simply by controlling the diets of laboratory animals, scientists have brought on, halted, and even reversed just about every ailment known. In other animals, again through diet alone, scientific workers have *prevented* these diseases.

The reason why diet has an influence over health is no mystery to modern science. Experts have identified more than fifty food elements necessary to life and health. About ten of these substances can be made within your body. The other forty or so must be obtained from the

[1] G.T. Wrench, M.D., *The Wheel of Health* (C.W. Daniel Company, Ltd., London, 1938).

food you eat. These figures are approximate, because from time to time other essential elements are discovered, and more are sure to be found in the future.

Unless your diet contains all of the forty or more necessary substances *in adequate amounts,* you're in trouble, or you will be sooner or later. The health of your heart, liver, brain, and all your other organs and that of your nerves, blood, bones and teeth depends on your getting a sufficient quantity of all the essential nutrients.

What are the forty magic food substances so important to your health and life?

Nutritionists divide the forty elements into five categories, according to their functions within the body. All the nutrients fall into one of these five basic categories: Protein, Carbohydrates, Fats, Vitamins or Minerals. Broadly, the function of each group is as follows:

Proteins are the materials from which your body is made.

Carbohydrates and *fats* furnish the energy to build and repair the body.

Vitamins and minerals carry on the tasks of building and repair of your body.

Although they are found in all natural foods, the leading sources of each of the five food categories are:

1. *Proteins*—foods of animal origin: meat, fish, eggs, and milk.
2. *Carbohydrates*—grains (wheat, corn, rice, etc.) and legumes (peas, beans, lentils).
3. *Fats*—meat, milk, nuts, seed foods.
4. *Vitamins*—fruits.
5. *Minerals*—vegetables.

Even though much of the nutritional good is refined or cooked out of American food, nearly everyone gets at least a smattering of each of the forty necessary elements. But in a great many diets, some of these are not present in sufficient quantities to protect health.

Not only is the typical American diet often short of some needed elements, but it also contains too much of one of the food categories, carbohydrate. This energy food is not required in the high quantities often consumed. The excess is stored by the body in the form of fat, resulting in the increasingly common condition of being overweight.

The "carbo-holic" who fills up on bulky carbohydrates —often refined ones, at that—usually does so at the expense of other more-needed foods. In spite of his full stomach and bloated body, he may be slowly starving to death.

Decades after McCarrison and others proved beyond doubt the connection between cooked and refined foods and poor health, years after nutritional researchers explained the reasons behind the proof, most of America is still looking elsewhere for the causes of disease.

To be sure, other factors besides diet enter into the picture. But it's hard to understand why the cure and prevention of disease through food reform has been so sadly neglected. Apparently, the facts about diet and health are little-known or appreciated; otherwise, the nutrition-robbing practices of cooking and refining would be far less common.

SUMMARY

The twin evils of cooking and refining rob our foods of the natural nutrients needed to build and protect health.

nine

Eat 'Em Alive

Man is the only creature who cooks his food. All the food that wild animals consume is eaten in raw form.

Man, until quite late in his evolution, also lived entirely on foods that were uncooked. Back in his prehuman days, during his sixty million years as a tree-dwelling primate, he lived on fresh raw fruit, nuts, and leaves. After he climbed down from the trees and began to augment his diet with meat and vegetables, they too were devoured uncooked.

We know that many ages elapsed before primitive man learned to kindle a fire. We know man invented cooking utensils only a few thousand years ago. The extensive use of cooked foods is an aberration of only the comparatively recent past, and it has not altered mankind's deep-rooted requirements for certain nutritional substances abundantly present in raw foods, which are reduced or entirely missing from foods that are cooked.

The heat of cooking damages or destroys various important elements present in all raw foods. Vitamins, for instance, are extremely delicate substances, easily affected by heat. The longer food is cooked, the more its vitamin content is depleted.

Cooking is particularly destructive to Vitamin C, which is considered by many nutritionists as the most important of the vitamins. It is also the most fragile and is easily damaged by cooking heat.

But a plentiful supply of Vitamin C is tremendously important to your health. This substance helps build healthy teeth and gums and is needed by most of your internal organs, including your heart and circulatory system.

A shortage of Vitamin C has been linked to cancer by some researchers. Comparing the blood of healthy people with the blood of cancer patients disclosed that the cancer sufferers were markedly deficient in Vitamin C. Comparing guinea pigs suffering from scurvy (the Vitamin C deficiency disease) with healthy guinea pigs showed that those deficient in Vitamin C were far more vulnerable to cancer, and that they developed it sooner.

Minerals, as well as vitamins, can suffer damage from the heat of cooking.

The most important mineral, in the judgment of a majority of nutritionists, is calcium. Cooking, in the opinion of many experts, tends to render calcium insoluble, thus making it less readily able to be assimilated by the body. What your body can't assimilate, it can't use. Even when enough calcium for your needs is present in your diet, your body is cheated of needed nutrition if cooking has affected the mineral's solubility.

Possible consequences of calcium shortage are described in *The Modern Family Health Guide,* edited by Morris Fishbein, former editor of the *Journal of the American Medical Association.* "A calcium deficiency may be involved in the cause of so-called degenerative diseases—

those diseases involving a loss in the power of functioning of any part of the body—such as hardening of the arteries . . . disorders of the heart . . . and blood vessels." [1]

The heat of cooking harms not only Vitamin C and calcium, but also other vitamins and minerals. Vitamins and minerals lost in cooking can't help you build your health. Plenty of uncooked foods in your diet will help to protect your body against the onslaught of disease.

Just as important to your body, though not so well-publicized as vitamins and minerals, is another group of food substances: enzymes. There are about six hundred and fifty different kinds of enzymes, each with its own specific functions within your system.

Without enzymes in your body to help the other food elements carry on their work, your life could not continue. If somehow the enzymes were suddenly removed from your body, you would die instantly.

Enzymes can be easily obtained, for they are found plentifully in all foods—vegetable or animal. However, the heat of cooking completely destroys them. Any heat slightly above body temperature (98°) quickly kills all enzymes. While vitamins and minerals can withstand some degree of heat without total destruction, enzymes can't withstand even a little heat. Raw foods contain a plentitude of enzymes, cooked foods none whatever.

By now you are probably asking "What about people who never eat raw foods? How do they stay alive without enzymes?"

They make their own. Like all other plants and animals, man manufactures enzymes within his cells. So everyone has two sources of enzymes, those which have been made in the cells of the substances he eats, and those made by his own cells.

[1] New York: Doubleday & Company, Inc., 1959.

But the person who eats cooked foods exclusively is totally dependent on his body for the production of enzymes. The raw-food eater makes things easier for his body. The more enzymes obtained from raw food, the less the body needs to manufacture.

Getting enzymes from food sources becomes particularly important as you grow older, because as you age, your body's enzyme-making apparatus may become less efficient, and enzyme production may diminish.

Cooking is popular because, among other reasons, cooked food keeps longer. It is the living enzymes in food that cause it to spoil. Killing the enzymes makes food last longer.

To provide your body with an abundance of needed vitamins, minerals, and enzymes, a generous portion of your food intake should be raw. The rule we Prohaskas try to follow is "50% raw food." If at least half your intake consists of an ever-changing variety of raw foods, you are pretty sure to get at least a fairly good supply of all the highly necessary vitamins, minerals, and enzymes.

All fruits and most vegetables can and should be eaten raw. Perhaps you often enjoyed a piece of sweet, juicy, raw fruit as a child but have gotten away from the raw-fruit habit as you got older. If so, I urge you to rediscover the taste treats of ripe, sweet, juicy, tender fruits.

Apples, pears, peaches, cherries, grapes, bananas, berries, various kinds of melon, citrus fruits like oranges, and many other fruits are all delicious raw. Instead of refined and cooked desserts, try finishing off meals with health-building raw fruit. Eat all you want without feeling guilty. Fruits are low in calories, which produce added weight. Never remove edible skins from fruit, for most of the vitamins and minerals lie near the surface. When you peel these foods, you cut away the most nourishing part.

Moreover, many vegetables can and should be eaten un-cooked. If you have been neglecting vegetables in their raw form, you have still more taste treats in store.

The easiest and most pleasant way to eat raw vegetables is in a salad. Green leafy vegetables like lettuce, celery, parsley, spinach, dandelion greens, beet greens, chicory, collards, endive, escarole, or kale are delicious in a tossed salad. They should be enjoyed in raw, crisp, nourishing form, instead of cooked and soggy and depleted.

It is a shame to reduce the nutritive value of these foods by cooking, as many people do with spinach and some of the others. If you have never eaten raw spinach, you will probably be surprised by the way it tastes, which is not at all like cooked spinach. There's a big nutritional differ-ence too.

To a salad of green, leafy vegetables may be added non-leafy raw vegetables, such as cucumbers, peppers, onions, radishes, or tomatoes. (The tomato, though com-monly thought of as a vegetable, is really a fruit, but no matter what you call it, the nutritive value is high.)

There is no reason to waste time in laboriously cutting vegetables into small pieces. Larger chunks are chewier and lose fewer nutrients from exposure to air. Many of the ingredients need not even be cut, for they can be broken more quickly by hand.

If tough vegetables such as carrots or cabbage are added, they should be grated or shredded. This is easily done with the help of a simple metal gadget sold in va-riety or hardware stores. Food can be either grated or shredded by rubbing it against the tool's perforated sides. To protect your fingers, use rubber guards of the kind sold in stationary or office-supply stores.

Complete your healthful salad by adding vegetable oil and a little lemon juice or vinegar. If desired, herbs or spices may also be added for seasoning.

Never peel vegetables, for you will be throwing their

most nourishing part away. This applies even to potatoes, which should be baked without peeling and eaten skins and all.

You may be surprised to find how much enjoyment a raw-vegetable salad and dessert of raw fruit adds to a meal. Moreover these foods not only taste good, they are also *good for you.*

Nuts and peanuts, like the fruits and vegetables to which they are related, are also rich in vitamins, minerals, and enzymes and should always be eaten raw.

A variety of raw nuts is carried by most supermarkets. These can be purchased either shelled or unshelled, but are most nourishing if shelled just before being eaten.

Raw peanuts can't be found in most supermarkets. You can perhaps get them from a wholesaler of nuts, as I do. A wholesale house will probably be glad to sell you raw peanuts if you buy in fairly large quantities. I get our raw peanuts from a jobber, twenty pounds at a time. Another probable source is any storekeeper who displays a nut-roasting machine.

When buying peanuts, make sure you get those that are *raw.* Some peanuts have been blanched or boiled for a few minutes to remove their red skins before roasting.

Certain edible seeds are high in nutritive value, and these should also always be eaten raw. Sunflower, pumpkin, squash, and sesame seeds are sold by health-food dealers.

When you begin using raw foods, you will be wise to make your transition a gradual one. A sudden switch to increased raw-food consumption may irritate a digestive tract little accustomed to handling uncooked food. You could start by making raw foods 10% or 15% of your diet, and gradually work up to making them 50% of your diet.

In imitation of early man, some modern raw-food enthusiasts eat absolutely nothing that is cooked. One

West Coast nature boy, who practices the hobby of skin-diving, even eats fish raw. Upon catching a small fish with his hands, he devours it at once, live—bones and all.

You won't want to go this far, I am sure, nor will it be necessary. You can even get enough of the needed food elements on a diet consisting of some foods that have been cooked.

Peas, beans, lentils, potatoes, sweet potatoes, corn, beets, turnips, pumpkins, and squash are some of the vegetables you will prefer to cook before eating. But if you like, even some of these vegetables may be consumed raw. Tender, young fresh peas and corn possess a flavor deliciously different from that when cooked. The flavor of raw potatoes is enjoyed by some.

When you cook vegetables, use only a little water, and include the water when you serve them. Food cooked in water releases a large proportion of its vitamins and minerals into the cooking liquid. If the water is discarded, so are many of the remaining vitamins and minerals. Vegetables should either be served in their cooking water, or the liquid drunk separately, like a broth. For the same reason, the liquid in canned vegetables should never be thrown away. It also contains valuable nutrients which are a part of the total food. The same is true of the water in which meat or fish is cooked.

Many of the health-conscious, seeking the benefits in uncooked foods, take in extra quantities of nutrition by drinking the juices of raw fruits and vegetables. Extracting the juice from plant foods is done with the aid of a small juicing machine, of which there are many brands on the market.

In the juice lies the concentrated nourishment of the plant. The discarded pulp contains few nutrients. This part is largely indigestible cellulose, valuable mainly as bulk, to help keep the intestines performing regularly. You can get enough of this needed bulk by taking some of your fruits and vegetables in solid form.

Bulk which would be too much for the stomach to handle is assimilated with ease when liquified. In the form of juice, a large quantity of raw food can easily be handled at one time by the body. For example, take carrots, and you should frequently! Nutritionists consider carrots a good source of all the known vitamins and minerals. Just try eating half a dozen raw carrots at a sitting! But these six carrots, when run through a juicer, become just a small, easy-to-drink glass of juice. A larger glass of concentrated nourishment can be made by combining five or six carrots, five or six stalks of celery, and a handful of spinach.

Vegetables more often than fruits are the foods selected to make into juice, perhaps because many raw vegetables are harder to eat and more filling.

Raw fruit and vegetable juices are quickly and easily assimilated, taking only twenty minutes or so to leave the stomach. They can be eaten between meals without overtaxing your digestive system.

Fruit and vegetable juices lose nutritive value upon exposure to heat and air. Even ordinary room temperature or being left standing in an uncovered container reduces their food value. However, juices may be stored for some time with very little loss in nutritive value if placed in a sealed container and kept refrigerated. One test showed that, in carrot juice stored in this manner, the Vitamin C loss over a period of three days was only 7%. Since Vitamin C is probably the most fragile of nutrients, the other elements presumably deteriorated even less.

Juicers are sold by some department and small-appliance stores, as well as by health-food dealers. If you want a juicer, don't make the mistake of buying a liquifier or blender. A liquifier simply grinds fruits or vegetables, reducing them to a thick mixture made up of juice and pulp, but a juicer separates the juice from the pulp, and the latter can then be easily discarded.

The only way to get raw juice is by preparing it yourself. The kind of juices you should drink cannot be bought in most stores, although a few health-food stores do specialize in making these for you while you wait. Canned, bottled, or cartoned juices have been cooked or heat-treated for pasteurization. Frozen concentrates are heated to kill enzymes before being frozen.

One kind of juice provides an exception to the rule that raw fruit juice is not often available commercially. During the fall, apple cider can be bought in and near many apple-growing localities. Cider is just like the tasty and healthful juice you yourself could extract from apples. The cider mill's equipment is a king-size version of the triturator-press type of juicer you may use in your own home. However, cider is sometimes preserved by pasteurizing or by the addition of chemicals. Such tampering is unnecessary except for preservation, so make sure the cider you buy is fresh, and free from preservatives.

By consuming in raw form whatever foods you can enjoy uncooked, you will be taking a big step toward attaining health and longevity.

Summary

To gain the health benefits of food's natural nutrients, make sure at least half of your total food intake is in raw, uncooked form, from fruits, vegetables, fruit and vegetable juices, nuts or peanuts, and seed foods, such as sunflower seeds.

ten

The Staff of Death

In stealing health-building elements from your foods, refining is cooking's partner in crime.

Were food refinement limited to a few seldom-used products, little harm would result, but the foods that have been devitalized are the ones we eat in the greatest quantities. Refined foods make up about *50% of the present-day American diet.* Half of the food sold in groceries and supermarkets has been partially or wholly stripped of its nutrients. The main offenders are products made of white flour and white sugar.

White bread, rolls, buns, biscuits, cakes, cookies, muffins, doughnuts, pastries, pies, pancakes, waffles, crackers, pizza, macaroni, spaghetti, noodles, and other white-flour products have been deprived of the greater part of their original nutritive value.

When I pass the shelves loaded with white bread in a supermarket, I always feel appalled that these loaves will be taken home by innocent buyers who have been hoodwinked into believing that this mock food is the staff of life.

Of even less nutritional value than white flour is white sugar, which has had virtually 100% of its nutritional elements removed.

Even those persons who never add a grain of sugar to their food will be hard put to avoid this lethal substance. Candy, ice cream, chewing gum, soft drinks, and many other commonly used treats are heavily loaded with refined sugar. Added to this deadly deluge are jams, jellies, canned fruits, dessert mixes, and many of the white-flour products previously mentioned.

Inasmuch as food refinement removes nutritional substances that are vitally necessary to our diets, why is this process perpetrated on an unsuspecting public?

In the case of white flour, this refinement acts as a preservative. Flour keeps indefinitely, without spoiling, when stripped of its most nutritional part, the germ. Deprived also of other nutrients, it then has little appeal to insects, so can more easily be kept free from insect infestation during shipping and storage. Thus, the miller, distributor, and baker are all insured against loss, and the fellow who then needs the insurance is the consumer.

Sugar is refined for a different reason. Sugar refiners are pandering to man's instinctive craving for sweetness, which is older than man himself. Man's forerunner, the ape, lived on foods which grew plentifully in trees. Even after he was forced to move to the ground, the ape-man did not lose his taste for fruit.

Fruit is replete with the vitamins so important to good health and long life, and it is the ripest, sweetest fruits which are the richest in vitamins. Those humans who regularly ate sweet fruit, with its health-building elements, were most fit to survive and reproduce. Thus a liking for sweets has been handed down to us, and, if anything, strengthened by the passing of time.

But there is a vast difference between natural plant

sugars and the artificial refined product, white sugar. The sugar in fruit (and in certain sweet vegetables, including sugar cane, from which white sugar is made) is in highly diluted form and accompanied, in correct proportions, by the vitamins and minerals necessary to its proper utilization within the body. But in the manufacture of sugar, the refining process extracts only the sweetness and leaves behind all the original nutrients.

In the milling of flour, 30% of the wheat grain is removed (the germ and the bran), and this is the most nutrition-laden part. What happens to all this rich concentration of vital food elements? It is considered scrap, fit only for livestock, which thus fare better than humans. Just how much better is detailed in *Saturday Review* by Science Editor John Lear.[1] Mr. Lear obtained his figures from the *Mill Feeds Manual*, published by the Millers National Federation through the Wheat Flour Institute in Chicago. Writes Mr. Lear:

This manual lists the contents of the wheat residue that goes into animal feeds after white flour has been milled for human consumption. It turns out that pigs get this much more of the vital nutrients in the whole wheat grain than people get in white flour:

21 times the Vitamin B_1
14 times the Vitamin B_2
16 times the Vitamin B_3
14 times the Vitamin B_6
4 times the pantothenic acid
11 times the folic acid
17 times the Vitamin E
2 times the choline
7 times the calcium
9 times the phosphorus

[1] *Saturday Review*, October 3, 1970.

12 times the magnesium
12 times the potassium
3 times the sodium
2 times the chromium
14 times the manganese
6 times the iron
42 times the cobalt
7 times the copper
12 times the zinc
3 times the molybdenum.

But not all of the nutritious waste of wheat ends up as animal fodder, for today some of these leavings find their way into health-food stores, where they are purchased by an informed minority of health-conscious humans.

In bygone days, bread was made from the entire wheat kernel, in which all of wheat's original elements were present in the proper proportion for digestion and assimilation. This kind of bread was eaten by your ancestors only a few generations ago, and is eaten today by the Hunzans, and by other unsophisticates who live in regions where modern flour-milling methods have not yet been introduced.

The refined bread eaten by today's Americans is mainly starch, which provides energy, but little else. The refining process has removed the greater share of nutrients, including most of the Vitamin E, which some nutritionists consider the vitamin most necessary to the body.

Still more Vitamin E is subtracted from the American diet by the refinement of various food oils. As a result of wholesale refinement, Vitamin E has been almost eliminated from our diet.

Noted nutritionist Adele Davis, in her book *Let's Get Well*, writes, "Our diets today contain only a fraction of the Vitamin E they did a century ago, and what little there is available is largely destroyed in cooking." [2] Miss Davis adds that our Vitamin E intake has dropped "from an estimated 150 units daily to a mere 8 to 15 units."

Some doctors and nutritionists feel that our greatly reduced intake of Vitamin E is primarily responsible for the great increase of heart disease.

Introduction of flour refinement coincides with the beginning of the American heart-disease epidemic. Refining of flour came into general use around 1910; about the same time, the incidence of coronary thrombosis began to increase. Previously, coronary thrombosis cases had been so rare that only a half dozen or so had been reported. Dr. Paul Dudley White, the famous heart specialist, says: ". . . when I graduated from medical school in 1911, I had never heard of coronary thrombosis, which is one of the chief threats to life in the United States and Canada today—an astonishing development in one's own lifetime!" [3]

The theory that a shortage of Vitamin E is at least partially responsible for heart ailments is strengthened by the work of two Canadian doctors, the Shute brothers. They have produced striking improvement in the conditions of thousands of heart-disease patients by administering large doses of Vitamin E. The Shutes' results have been matched by those of many other workers in various parts of the world.

In addition to its apparent connection with heart disease, lack of Vitamin E may also be a contributing factor to the onset of cancer. In an earlier chapter, I presented evidence which indicated that an insufficient supply of oxygen to the body's cells was related to the development

[2] Adelle Davis, *Let's Get Well* (Harcourt, Brace and World, Inc., New York, 1965).
[3] *Prevention*, December, 1969.

of cancer. Vitamin E has the power to carry extra oxygen
to the body's cells, and it could well be that when a
generous quantity of Vitamin E is present in the diet, the
development of cancer is inhibited.

You can help yourself live longer by eliminating white-
flour foods from your life and replacing them with Vitamin E-rich whole-grain products. Bread made from unrefined whole grain is available at many stores. If your
grocery or supermarket doesn't stock it, you can ask them
to order it from one of their suppliers.

Don't fall for come-ons that label bread as "wheat" or
"cracked wheat." Such imitation health foods are partially
made of white flour. Make sure the label on the bread you
buy reads "100% whole wheat."

Don't be fooled by "enriched" white-flour products.
Refining removes twenty or more known nutrients in
whole or in part, and enrichment returns only four of
these.

When you check bread labels, look for the words "stone
ground." Formerly, grain was ground slowly, between
large, flat stones. This method is still used in societies
more primitive than ours, but stone-grinding is too slow
for America's cost-conscious millers, who grind flour between high-speed steel rollers. The intense heat built up
by steel-grinding is yet another cause of damage to the
nutrients. However, a few producers of whole-wheat flour
still grind it in the old-fashioned way.

Whole-rye bread is excellent fare, if you can get it,
but most rye bread contains some white wheat flour.

A variety of whole-grain products other than breads
can be purchased from health-food dealers. If you feel
you can't live without delicacies like cookies and macaroni, eat the whole-grain kind, which you can at least
live *with*.

If there is no health-food store in your area, you can find the addresses of mail-order health-food dealers by looking in health magazines. Two such magazines are: *Prevention*, 33 East Minor Street, Emmaus, Pennsylvania 18049; and *Let's Live*, 444 North Larchmont Boulevard, Los Angeles, California 90004.

The health-food trade can also supply you with food oil, which has not had its Vitamin E depleted. And if, for insurance, you would like some extra Vitamin E, health-food dealers provide the vitamin concentrate in capsule form.

What has been said about the refining of wheat is largely true of other grains, such as rice and corn. These are also often refined before being packaged or before becoming a part of some other food product.

Most of the rice sold in this country is refined white rice. White rice is so lacking in food elements that, when it forms a principal part of the diet, the deficiency disease beri-beri is usually prevalent. Healthful, whole brown rice is carried by health-food dealers and by some super-markets.

Like white wheat flour, commercial cornmeal has been robbed of its germ, but in a few ground-corn products, the germ has not been removed. Look for the words "whole grain corn," or better still "stone-ground whole grain corn" on the label.

The grains from which most breakfast cereals are made have been greatly devitalized. Most of the so-called "ready to eat" breakfast cereals are really only ready to be thrown away.

Despite the nutritional weaknesses (or perhaps because of them) of breakfast cereals, they are well promoted. *Fortune* magazine reports: "In recent years, cereal companies have spent as much as fifteen cents of each dollar on advertising, more than double the spending rate of coffee roasters and soup canners, and nearly three times that of cake-mix producers." [4] Notwithstanding the manufacturers' overblown claims, analysis shows that most breakfast cereals are considerably lower in nutritional content than the grains from which they were produced. By the time corn, wheat, rice, and oats are flaked, puffed, shredded, or exploded, these products may have lost most of their food value.

In breakfast-cereal tests conducted at Distillation Products Industries, a division of Eastman Kodak Company in Rochester, New York, the loss of Vitamin E due to processing was found to be as high as 98%. In their report to the Federation for American Societies for Experimental Biology, Dr. David C. Herting and Miss Emma-Jane E. Drury stated that analysis of breakfast cereal grains showed Vitamin E losses as follows:

1. Rice—more than 70%.
2. Wheat—up to 92%.
3. Oats: About 95%.
4. Corn: Up to 98%.

Even whole grains come under attack by some nutritionists. According to these authorities, grains are, quite literally "for the birds," whose constitutions are better adapted to handling this class of food than are the physical systems of human beings.

The basis for the anti-grain theory is that man has not been a grain-eater for a long enough period of time. He began to use this kind of food only after he began to farm, so he has perhaps been eating grains only for a mere five thousand years. Evolutionarily speaking, this is a short time span—and quite possibly it is too soon for

[4] *Fortune,* December, 1967.

the human system to have fully adjusted to this type of food.

Wheat, in particular, is held in low esteem by some. Though wheat germ is considered an excellent health food, gluten, which forms the bulk of the wheat berry, is thought to be a contributor to various ills, among which is tooth decay.

But the pro-grain school musters good arguments in favor of grain-eating. Rather than trying to decide which side is right, or more right, I would suggest that you do as I do. Eat a moderate amount of whole grains, to get some of the good in this type of food, but don't eat enough to constitute an excess. In that way, you should be able to eat your cake (whole grain, of course) and have it too.

SUMMARY

Avoid nutritionally deficient white-flour foods, white rice, degerminated cornmeal products, and most breakfast cereals. Eat, instead, natural whole-grain foods.

eleven

The Un-Food

If white flour is bad, white sugar is even worse. At least a little nutrition is left in white flour, but with white sugar, nothing is left but pure, empty carbohydrate by the time the refining process has been completed.

True, this carbohydrate does produce energy, but it does so at great cost to your body. Refinement strips away virtually 100% of the nutrients in sugar. Gone are the minerals and vitamins originally in the sugar that are necessary for its oxidation. In order for sugar to be utilized, it must steal the required nutrients from your body. White sugar is the most foodless of all foods; it has become an "unfood" which takes from your body more than it contributes. It is now only an energy-producer, and a highly inefficient one at that.

"The increase in the consumption of sugar is the most outstanding dietetic perversion of the age," writes Macpherson Lawrie, M.D., in his book *Nature Hits Back.* "Apart from any other consideration, it upsets the whole balance of nutrition. Sugar is a fuel, and today we take into our system this purely fuel food in amounts sufficient to shatter every dietetic principle and law. Our digestive glands and organs may be adaptable, but it is impossible to believe that during the last hundred years our physiological processes have so changed as to enable our bodies to deal normally with an excess of fuel so staggering." [1]

In its destructive effects on the health of the heart, white sugar rivals white flour.

Dr. John Yudkin of the University of London, a leading scientist, has come up with strong evidence that an excess of sugar in the diet is a cause of heart trouble. His studies show an unmistakable connection between heart disease and the heavy consumption of sugar. His findings have been backed up by the work of many other medical investigators, and statistical evidence reinforces the theory that links refined sugar to heart trouble. Moreover, those countries which use most white sugar also suffer the most heart disease.

In our country, the rise of heart disease has paralleled the increase in sugar consumption. In 1900, before heart disease had become widespread, our consumption of sugar was only about ten pounds per capita. By 1935, the figure had increased to one hundred pounds per person a year. Today, it is well over this amount.

Were the practice of food refinement linked only to heart trouble and cancer, this surely would be enough to justify its abolition, but food processing also produces further baneful consequences. One is its effect on teeth. Tooth decay, though less serious than some of the other diseases connected with food refinement is today America's most common ailment. Ninety-eight percent of our

[1] Macpherson Lawrie, M.D., *Nature Hits Back* (Kingswood, England: Surrey World's Work, 1960).

population has been affected by some degree of tooth decay. One out of eight Americans has lost all of his teeth.

A *Science Digest* article says: "Teeth are decaying faster than dentists can be trained to fix them. If all 94,000 practicing members of the American Dental Association worked at top speed repairing teeth alone, there still would be six new cavities forming for every one filled."

This wasn't always the case. The teeth of early man, who lived on a naturally balanced diet of raw, unrefined foods, were practically free from decay. P. O. Pederson of the Danish Royal Dental College estimates prehistoric European tooth decay in adults at only 1%.

The examination of thirty thousand Egyptian mummies revealed no tooth decay except among the luxury classes, whose "superior" diets, much like ours today, rendered them vulnerable to tooth trouble.

Today, in those parts of the world where a variety of food is eaten in its natural state, tooth decay is still either rare or nonexistent. The classic study of tooth health in primitive cultures was made by Dr. Weston Price. Dr. Price traveled thousands of miles in forty-five countries to study both primitive people and those who live in modern societies. He examined people with good teeth and compared their living habits with those of people with poor teeth.

Dr. Price found good teeth wherever he found the natives were eating natural, whole foods; wherever the populace ate unnatural, refined foods, he found bad teeth.

A refined diet that is short in minerals forces the body to borrow the elements it needs from the bones and teeth. Bones become softer and more easily broken, and teeth decay.

To make matters worse, a refined diet also attacks the teeth from without. As soon as sugar enters the mouth, certain acids begin to form. These acids quickly attack tooth enamel. Even the residues from wholesome foods can, to a lesser extent, produce potentially harmful mouth acids.

Those people who eat or snack frequently manage to expose their teeth to decay around the clock, even though some of the between-meal treats consist of only a cough drop or a soft drink.

To protect your teeth, cleanse them thoroughly immediately after you eat or drink anything except plain water. Brushing provides the most thorough cleaning. However, toothpaste, with its gritty polishes, can wear away the tooth enamel you are striving to keep, so brush with plain water. Save on toothpaste, and save your teeth.

When you can't brush, a thorough rinsing may be almost as beneficial. Where school playgrounds are equipped with drinking fountains, tooth decay among pupils has been found to be less than where drinking facilities are not provided. The factor that makes the difference is apparently that when food is consumed before and after school and during recess, the residue remaining on the teeth is more likely to be rinsed away.

"How about early man?" you may ask. "He didn't own a toothbrush." No, but the food he ate cleaned his teeth for him. His coarse raw diet contained a built-in cleaning action. Raw fruits and vegetables are the toothbrushes that nature provides for us. Such foods helped keep the teeth of early man in good condition, and the minerals in raw fruits and vegetables helped to maintain the teeth from within. When you can't brush, it's still a good idea to finish your meal with a hard, firm fruit or vegetable.

Dr. Geoffrey L. Slack, a British dentist, made a two-year study of apple-eating as a method of cleaning teeth. One group of children was given unpeeled apple slices after every meal or snack. The control group received none. The apple-eaters developed only half as much tooth decay as the control group, and only one-third as much gum trouble.

At the same time a deficient diet causes *visible* damage to teeth, it also inflicts *invisible* injury on other parts of the body. Once your teeth develop cavities, it is already *past* the time for you to correct your diet.

Sugar like alcohol, that other pure carbohydrate, is not really a food, but a drug. The sugar drunkard may find it difficult to swear off his habit. He may even suffer withdrawal symptoms something like those experienced by the alcoholic who is trying to "dry out." If you feel the need to add a sweetener to some of your foods, perhaps even for a tapering-off period, healthful, unrefined sugars can be had.

One such nonharmful sweetener which can be used in place of sugar is blackstrap molasses, the product that remains after sugar has been refined. Blackstrap molasses is not a substitute for sugar. Sugar itself is the substitute, and a sorry one it is. Blackstrap molasses is everything that sugar is not, so if you are trying to kick the white-sugar habit, hurry down to your supermarket or your health-food store and get some blackstrap molasses.

Honey is another nutritious sweetener, for in gathering nectar from flowers, the honey bee also gathers vitamins and minerals.

Most shoppers select a light-colored, "pure-looking" honey, but the darker honeys contain more nutritional value. The best honey is raw and unstrained. Most honey sold in stores has been heated during extraction, then strained. Both processes subtract nutrients. Raw, unstrained honey can be bought from health-food dealers. Another source of such honey is a bee-keeper, provided he can be persuaded to extract some of his honey for you without heating it and to leave it unstrained.

Maple sugar is yet another wholesome sweetener. But when you buy maple sugar or maple syrup, be sure to read the fine print on the label to make sure that the product is 100% maple sugar, without any white sugar added.

What about raw sugar, the sweetener used in some foods sold by health-food dealers? Though less devitalized than white sugar, raw sugar is not a complete food, for this product has undergone some refinement. It is best for the truly health-minded to avoid it. Plenty of good wholesome sweets are available.

Another fooler on labels is the term "brown sugar." Brown sugar is used instead of white by some health-conscious persons who have the mistaken notion that the deeper color indicates the presence of nutritional substances. However, brown sugar has undergone even more processing than white sugar. Most of the brown color comes from the bone charcoal used in the refining process, not from the smattering of remaining minerals.

The careful reading of labels will help you eliminate white sugar and other harmful sugars from your diet. When you study the labels, don't be fooled by devitalized sugar masquerading under aliases such as "dextrose" or "glucose." It is deadly under any name.

Also on the unhealthful list are the various artificial sweeteners (as if sugar itself weren't artificial!). Like sugar, these substances are completely foodless and should be avoided like the poisons they are.

Go easy even on the three healthful sweeteners, blackstrap molasses, honey, and maple sugar. Though high in nutrients, they are all concentrated sugars, which are not like the diluted sugars found in fruits and vegetables. Too much of any concentrated sugar can give you an overdose of carbohydrate, an element you need only in limited quantities.

Actually, adding extra sugar, even the wholesome kind,

to your diet is unnecessary. Natural-food eaters get plenty of unrefined sugar in their diets, for fruits and certain vegetables provide them with all the sugar they need.

Summary

Avoid white sugar and foods containing white sugar. If you desire a sweetener, use blackstrap molasses, honey, or maple sugar.

To protect your teeth, cleanse the teeth by brushing with plain water or by rinsing the mouth immediately after eating or drinking anything except water.

twelve

Have a Heart

Two other heart-harming, artery-attacking modern mock-foods are salt and hydrogenated fats.

The salt that nature puts into food is in the form of *sodium*, one of the minerals necessary to life. But table salt, which is procured from inorganic salt deposits, is merely a flavoring substance and has no food value whatsoever.

Man not only has no need for this inert material, but its use is also decidedly harmful. Too much table salt in the diet has been proved to be one cause of colds. More serious is the effect of salt on heart and artery health. Excessive salt-eating has been shown to contribute to high blood pressure, a forerunner to heart trouble. This is why doctors forbid salt in the diet of those who suffer from high blood pressure.

Earlier, man did without salt, as do many primitive people today who are isolated from civilization. But if you try to give up salt, you will find it almost impossible, even if you throw away your salt shaker. Salt finds its way into food more often than any other additive: Bread, cheese, and canned vegetables are only a few of the foods which contain salt.

Among the foods that contain salt are commercial baby foods. Yet the salting of strained meats and vegetables is unnecessary, for infants have not yet acquired the salt habit. The manufacturers of these foods are appealing to mothers, who often sample baby foods. Though better for baby's health, unsalted food would taste bland to the mother, so children are given an early start on the road to high blood pressure.

Most people who give up salt miss its taste at first, but they soon begin to enjoy the true flavor of food, which has hitherto been masked by salt. If flavoring is desired, it can be added by using lemon juice and herbs. Oregano, sage, basil, and curry are a few of the herbs which add flavor to food without harming health.

In addition to the refining of food, food processors have discovered still another way of tampering with food. This process is called hydrogenation.

Hydrogenation differs from refining in that it takes nothing away from food. Instead, it does damage by altering the composition of food. This affects the oil in foods of vegetable origin. The oils in many of the foods now on sale at your supermarket have undergone hydrogenation.

Unhydrogenated, the oils naturally contained in vegetable foods are proportionately high in the unsaturated fatty acids that are indispensable to many bodily processes. But hydrogenation changes the proportions of vegetable oils so that the saturated oils are predominant. Saturated oils or fats are believed by many authorities to contribute to the formation of cholesterol, a clogging substance, in the arteries. Cholesterol is the villain responsible for many heart attacks and strokes.

Why do food processors practice hydrogenation? Because saturated fats keep better than the unsaturated ones. The natural unsaturated oil in a jar of peanut butter may become rancid. The food would then have to be recalled from the supermarket at a loss to one of the handlers. But if the processor of the peanut butter has taken the precaution of hydrogenating the oil, the product can sit on the grocer's shelf without spoiling for a long time. Then the processor is happy, the distributor is happy, and the grocer is happy. And the customer is also happy because he never brings home a jar of peanut butter that is rancid.

Hydrogenation of vegetable oils helps the food business in yet another way. It turns liquid oils into hard fats, and thereby enables processors to create margarine and solid vegetable shortenings.

The chemists don't know everything that happens when vegetable oils are hydrogenated. No one knows exactly what effect this causes inside the human body. What the chemists *do* know is that hydrogenation helps food processors make money.

You can avoid hydrogenated foods by checking the labels on products you buy. If the fat in a food has been hydrogenated, the label must say so.

The same warnings as those against hydrogenated vegetable fats are applicable to all animal fats, which are predominantly of the saturated kind. These fats have been hydrogenated or saturated in the bodies of the animals from which they came. The fat found in meat, milk, and eggs is the kind which many authorities believe contributes to the formation of arterial cholesterol. Therefore, the cholesterol-conscious go easy on fatty meats like beef and pork and eat more fish and poultry, which are lower in fat.

Cholesterol can also be avoided by substituting skim

milk for whole milk. Skim milk contains all of the food value of whole milk except for the fat and the Vitamin A which accompanies the fat. Butter, the source of which is the fat part of milk, is high in saturated fat, as is cheese.

Whether or not animal fats cause arterial cholesterol formation is, at present, controversial. Some authorities consider animal fats guilty, while others feel that no convincing scientific evidence of this guilt exists. Until the question is resolved one way or the other, it would be prudent to keep animal-fat consumption moderate.

However, *vegetable* fat of the *unsaturated* type is a daily necessity, not only for its reputed attribute of reducing blood-cholesterol levels, but also for its highly essential unsaturated fatty acids.

As essential as a certain amount of vegetable fat is, a large quantity of it should never be taken at one meal. If a large amount of fat is taken at one meal, digestion of the other foods is hindered. Fat covers the other foods and inhibits penetration of digestive fluids.

Fats are not digested until they reach the intestines. Carbohydrate digestion begins in the mouth, and proteins digest in the stomach, so when carbohydrate and protein foods are covered by fats, digestion of them is hindered. For this reason, fried foods are extremely hard to digest. When food is fried in fat or oil, each particle becomes coated with fat.

Nuts and peanuts should always be eaten raw, not roasted, for roasting, as it is called, is really boiling in oil. Potato chips, french fries, and similar snack foods have all been cooked in oil.

Foods eaten cooked are best baked, broiled, or boiled. Eggs are most easily digested when poached.

Have a heart; help your health. Avoid salt and hydrogenated fats and forsake fried foods.

SUMMARY

Avoid salt. Use lemon juice and herbs if you desire flavoring.

Avoid hydrogenated fats. Eat less animal fat, more vegetable fat. Avoid fried foods.

thirteen

Fleshies and Veggies

Thus far we have talked mostly about four of the five basic food categories: vitamin, mineral, carbohydrate, and fat. The one remaining category is protein, the substance from which the body is built.

The body doesn't store protein as it does most of the other elements, so it must obtain a fresh supply daily.

The best, most-complete protein is generally considered to be that of animal origin: meat, fish, eggs, and milk. A secondary source of protein is from vegetables: legumes (peas, beans, lentils), grains, and nuts. This brings us to the subject of meat-eating versus vegetarianism.

Vegetarians believe in getting their protein entirely from vegetable sources. Vegetarians avoid meat because they claim that it is filled with poisonous toxins, which are the end products of animal metabolism. Meat, says the anti-flesh faction, putrefies in the human intestines and damages the kidneys and liver.

To support their anti-meat stand, vegetarians use the evolution argument. In his prehuman form, as an ape, man ate no meat. For sixty million years, he thrived as a vegetarian. Only when he descended to the ground did man begin to add animal foods to his diet. Man is not a natural meat-eater, argue the vegetarians, and so his constitution has never adjusted to the feeding habits forced on it by evolutionary conditions.

The advocates of meat-eating oppose this argument by saying that man has had two million years to adapt to animal foods. Moreover, they claim that man has even become dependent upon a diet containing animal foods.

There are various sects among non-meat-eaters. In addition to the strict vegetarians, there are those who believe in a limited use of animal products. "Lacto-vegetarians" avoid meat, but use milk. "Lacto-ovo-vegetarians" also do not eat meat, but use both milk and eggs.

Who is right? The fleshies, the strict veggies, the ovos, or the lacto-ovos?

A study of the eating habits of the healthy and long-lived doesn't produce conclusive evidence in favor of any group. Among those Gallup surveyed, only about 2% were vegetarians. This is perhaps the same proportion of vegetarians to be found among the general population. The Hunzans could almost be called non-meat-eaters. Since the Hunzans can't afford to waste egg- and milk-producing animals by killing them for meat, they eat meat only on special occasions. However, they regularly partake of animal products in the form of goat milk and cheese and eggs.

Some individual vegetarians have achieved impressive health and longevity records. George Bernard Shaw and Upton Sinclair are among those who lived long and healthful lives.

Perhaps all this only shows that man can be healthy on

any diet, especially one that contains whole and natural foods. Whether or not animal foods are included may be of a minor consideration.

Does science have anything to say regarding the relative merits of meat-eating as opposed to vegetarianism?

Science has discovered one good reason for using animal protein rather than vegetable protein. All protein, it has been found, is composed of amino acids. The body converts these acids into protein it can use. Although the body is able to make some amino acids, there are at least ten which can't be made internally and must, therefore, be obtained from the food we eat.

Some protein foods do not contain all ten of the essential amino acids. Since the body can't properly utilize protein unless all ten are present in sufficient quantities at the same time, these incomplete proteins are not efficient body-builders. One can gorge on protein foods, but if they contain only eight or nine of the ten essential amino acids in the quantities needed, the body will not profit as much as it would from a complete protein food, which was rich in all ten of the essential amino acids.

Which are the complete proteins, and which the incomplete? For the most part, the complete proteins are those found in animal foods, the incomplete those in plant foods. Meat, fish, eggs, and milk contain complete proteins; nuts, grains, and legumes, incomplete proteins.

In view of the findings regarding amino acids, it would appear that man has grown dependent on having some animal foods in his diet. Strict vegetarians, who eschew all foods of animal origin, find it difficult to meet their protein needs. If they remain in good health, it would appear that they manage to do so in spite of their eating habits. Perhaps their other health practices make up for what they lose by avoiding animal foods.

Nothing is wrong with plant protein except that it does not contain all of the essential amino acids in sufficient quantities. If the missing amino acids were provided, these proteins would be fully usable. This is exactly what happens when a complete animal protein is added to a meal that contains only incomplete vegetable protein. Then, all the protein ingested by the body becomes complete. The missing amino acids are added by those in the complete protein. Only a little of the complete animal protein is enough to compensate for the missing amino acids in the plant protein. Animal foods are so rich in all the essential amino acids that they are able to compensate for those that are lacking in the plant foods. When you combine a portion of animal protein with one or more plant proteins in the same meal, all the protein becomes complete. All ten amino acids are now present in sufficient quantities, and all of the protein eaten is now usable.

Therefore, it is important to get some complete protein at every meal. When you eat incomplete protein, such as that found in grains, legumes, and nuts, be certain to include a portion of meat, fish, milk (or cheese), or eggs at the same meal. In this way, you will get full benefit from all the protein in the meal.

The opinion of the majority of nutritionists concurs with my rating of protein completeness. But this is by no means a unanimous one. Individual experts often disagree on whether a given protein food should be classed as complete or incomplete. Some authority or other will argue whether or not the protein found in just about any plant can be considered complete.

Many nutritionists consider the protein in soybeans to be of the complete type. However, despite the fact that the soybean contains all the essential aminos, it is quite low in two of them, tryptophan and methionine. For this reason, some nutritionists consider soy protein incomplete.

The same disputes exist with regard to nuts, peanuts, and grains. Most experts rank these foods with the second-class or incomplete proteins, but some authorities can be found who feel that they are complete.

Among the foods that are not commonly eaten, the plant world has given us three sources of protein that are considered complete. These are sunflower seeds, wheat germ, and brewer's yeast, all three of which are available from health-food dealers.

What about the claims made by vegetarians—that meat putrefies in the digestive tract and that it contains toxins capable of damaging the liver and kidneys? Is scientific evidence available pro or con on this matter? Experiments indicate that there is some validity in the vegetarians' charges.

Science says the vegetarians are right about meat putrefying in the lower digestive tract. Mitchell and Hamilton, two researchers, name eggs and meat as the protein foods which putrefy most readily. They rate vegetable proteins second, and milk protein third. Not only is milk protein the least putrefactive; it also renders the other proteins less so.

What about the reputed harmfulness of meat to the liver and kidneys? At the University of Michigan, Newburgh and Johnston compared the effects of various proteins on rats. A diet extremely high in liver and beef-muscle protein caused serious kidney damage. The same high proportion of protein derived from milk, wheat, or soybeans caused no harm.

Dr. Mann of the Mayo Foundation compared the consequences of ingesting meat protein and milk protein on dogs with severely damaged livers. The animals fed meat protein died within a few days, those on the same amount of milk protein lived for months. Dr. Mann attributed these findings to certain extractives that can be isolated from meat, but are missing from milk. When fed to dogs, these extractives caused even more damage than the meat alone.

So, there you have evidence that meat protein may be harmful to your kidneys and liver, especially when taken to excess.

All of the foregoing scientific information, it must be admitted, makes the lacto-vegetarians look good. Yet, in view of mankind's long history of flesh-eating, it is reasonable to hypothesize that he has possibly acquired a need for meat and/or fish. It is possible that some needed element or elements still undiscovered are present in flesh foods and lacking in other foods, even milk and eggs.

After weighing all the evidence, I have adopted a middle-of-the-road policy. I eat meat and fish to get some of whatever is good in flesh foods, but in order not to overburden my body with toxins, I eat these flesh foods in limited quantities. With this compromise, I hope to live in harmony with both of the groups in my evolutionary background, the early vegetarians and the later meat-eaters. Moreover, while partaking lightly of meat and fish, I indulge more heavily in milk, the least putrefactive of all protein foods.

A final word about the cooking of meat, which is one food that should never be eaten raw. Raw meat, sometimes eaten in "cannibal" sandwiches, may contain harmful bacteria.

Certain foods of animal origin are unacceptable for the health-seeker because they contain poisons harmful to the health.

Meat products like bologna, frankfurters, sausage, cold

cuts, and most canned meats have been treated with chemical preservatives that can be damaging to the health of the user.

Fish from inland waters sometimes contain harmful chemical pollutants, for many of our streams, rivers, and lakes are subject to poisonous pollution. The flesh of fish caught in such waters is often found to contain dangerously high levels of harmful chemicals.

Because shellfish are usually harvested from coastal waters near the mouths of rivers, they are also subject to contamination. Since there is the possibility that these otherwise acceptable foods may be polluted, the health-minded should avoid fish from inland waters and shellfish such as clams, oysters, lobsters, and shrimp.

My animal-protein program, in a few words, is more milk, fewer flesh foods, and no poisoned proteins.

SUMMARY

To derive full benefit from the incomplete protein foods in your meals, eat some complete animal protein food— meat, fish, milk, or eggs—at every meal.

Eat meat and eggs, the most highly putrefactive proteins, in moderation. Use milk, the least putrefactive protein, in greater quantities than either eggs or meat.

Avoid "cold-meat products," such as bologna, frankfurters, sausage, cold cuts, and canned meats. Also avoid shellfish and fish from inland waters.

fourteen

Unforbidden Fruit

To the new disciple of healthful diet, the going may seem difficult. Since so many commonly used foods are on the forbidden list, the convert may begin to think that very little is left that he can eat safely. Actually, there is no end to the healthful replacements for unhealthful foods.

Cold-meat products are easy to skip, what with the availability of a wide variety of fresh meats and ocean fish and cheese and eggs. All fruits and vegetables can still be eaten, and those which should be eaten raw actually taste better that way. Whole-grain breads have more flavor than those made from refined flour.

Blackstrap molasses, honey, and maple sugar sweeten as well as white sugar and add flavor at the same time. Sugar-loaded soft drinks can be supplanted by fruit and vege-table juices or milk. Devitalized breakfast cereals may be replaced by the unprocessed ones that are available from health-food dealers. For extra nourishment, wheat germ may be sprinkled on these wholesome cereals. Breakfast is also a good time to enjoy fruit.

Healthful desserts are easily concocted, to replace unsuitable ones like pastries and ice cream.

One simple, yet tasty, dessert is a mixture of raisins and raw peanuts in the proportions you prefer. A slightly fancier dessert is a mixture of raw nuts, raw peanuts, and honey. Another easily made dessert consists of raw, pitted dates which have raw nut meats replacing the missing pits.

Frozen fruit-juice concentrates, such as those made from oranges or pineapples, are excellent replacements for ice cream. Instead of being thinned with water, the concentrate is eaten as is with a spoon.

The housewife with imagination can dream up many other healthful desserts. Perhaps the finest dessert a housewife can put on her table is a bowl of assorted fruit.

Raw fruits also make the best snacks. Rather than snacking on unhealthful foods like potato chips, it is better to munch raisins, dates, figs, or other raw fruits.

Another healthful snack, one which is greatly enjoyed by children, consists of ice cubes made by freezing fruit juice.

If you must have snacks of something more filling than fruit, I suggest raw nut meats, raw peanuts, or raw seed foods, such as sunflower seeds.

It is not always easy to get all the vitamins and minerals you need, even from raw, unrefined fare. The food you buy has often been subjected to nutritional depletion in various ways. Much of it is grown in overworked, impoverished soil, which has been fertilized chemically instead of with natural fertilizers. Food also loses nutrients while it is being shipped and stored.

You can boost your vitamin and mineral intake by eating special foods that you can obtain from health-food dealers. These uncommon products are extra-rich in important vitamins and minerals. Brewer's yeast, desiccated liver, bone meal, kelp, dolomite, and acerola contain vitamins and minerals in a high concentration. From whence come these exotic-sounding viands? All are derived from natural-food sources.

Brewer's yeast, which consists of microscopic yeast plants, is abundant in all the vitamins of the important B family.

Desiccated liver is another rich source of all the B Vitamins. In addition, some experts conjecture that liver contains one or more yet-to-be-isolated nutrients which are virtually unobtainable from other foods. But getting people to eat liver can be difficult. Some people don't like its taste, and even those who do, hardly care to eat it daily. Moreover, most housewives wouldn't want to cook liver every day. These objections are easily overcome by taking desiccated-liver tablets. Desiccated liver is extra high in nutritive value because it has been prepared with very little heat.

Powdered bone meal consists of the ground shank bones of young beef cattle, and it contains various minerals in the proportions required by the teeth and bones.

Powdered kelp is made by drying certain ocean-growing seaweed. Kelp is mineral-rich because the oceans contain dissolved minerals in a high proportion. Every mineral and a dozen different vitamins are found in kelp.

Dolomite, a substance mined from the earth, is rich in calcium and other minerals. When you begin to use dolomite, you will probably be subject to slight diarrhea for a few days. This is the result of the natural cleansing action of the high magnesium content of dolomite. This is a harmless symptom which will soon disappear.

Another health food which will help keep you well-nourished is the acerola berry, the world's richest natural source of Vitamin C. Its Vitamin C content is five thousand times more potent than fresh orange juice. Vitamin C derived from the acerola berry is available in tablet form.

Keeping the body supplied with sufficient Vitamin C is not an easy task. The body needs large quantities of this important element, and it is so rapidly used up, or excreted through urine or perspiration, that a fresh supply is needed several times a day.

High in Vitamin C are citrus fruits such as oranges and grapefruit and their juice, but it isn't always convenient to use these sources. At such times, Vitamin C tablets come in handy. These tablets make it easy for you to keep your cells saturated with Vitamin C.

You may wonder why man's system is so dependent on frequent doses of Vitamin C. We must take another of our trips backward through time for the probable answer. The ape quenched his thirst, not with water but with food. He ate enough juicy fruits and leaves to take care of his thirst. These same thirst-quenching habits have been observed in wild gorillas today. Zoologist George Schaller, an expert who has studied wild gorillas more closely than any other man, learned that these animals get all the liquids they need from food alone. Dr. Schaller says, "I have never seen gorillas drink in the wild."

The fruits and leaves with which the ape formerly satisfied his thirst were the very foods that were highest in Vitamin C content, so man's predecessor received frequent doses of this vitamin.

Early man must also have depended on fruits and leaves more than he did on drinking water to quench his thirst. Nature did not create man as a water-drinking animal. He does not possess the long snout of animals such as the horse or cow, which can easily drink from a pool or stream. Moreover, when early man was thirsty, drinking water wasn't always nearby. Therefore, it is logical to assume that man often quenched his thirst with the juicy fruits and green leafy foods that grew bountifully in his natural habitat. It was probably in this way that, over a span of many millions of years, we built up a need for frequent doses of Vitamin C.

Many persons who step up their vitamin C intake notice that they either suffer from fewer colds or avoid them entirely. In my own case, it was not until I added frequent consumption of Vitamin C to my other health habits that I became almost free from colds. I now sometimes go for years without getting a cold.

I start my daily Vitamin C intake upon arising, with a glass of fresh orange juice. Later, with breakfast, and again with lunch, I take a Vitamin C tablet. With dinner, which I like to eat just before I retire, I take another Vitamin C tablet. On many days, I also add a large, between-meals glass of juice from raw vegetables, which includes the juice of several green leafy vegetables that are high in Vitamin C content.

In view of the vital importance of vitamins and minerals to health and long life, many present-day nutritionists advocate extra measures to insure an adequate supply. In addition to a nutritional diet, the taking of vitamin and mineral supplements is recommended to compensate for possible dietary deficiencies.

Believers in food supplements in this country support a five hundred million dollar a year industry. This is called quackery by some, who contend that most people get all the vitamins and minerals they need from their normal diets.

However, many studies indicate otherwise. Test after test has shown that a high proportion of Americans are inadequately nourished. For example, in one survey of 169 people selected at random, 61% were found to be deficient in Vitamin C.

To help guard against possible deficiencies in the diet, it seems a sensible precaution for the average American to take daily multiple vitamin and mineral supplements in tablet form. This will help bring his intake nearer to the needed level.

One risk of using vitamin and mineral supplements is that people sometime depend on them and neglect their diet. It is a mistake to eat depleted foods and then try to compensate for deficiencies by gulping down supplements. Supplements can never substitute for the proper foods. Whole foods, just as they are created by nature, are the ones to which our bodies have adapted during evolution. Supplements should be just that—supplements to a diet already loaded with a wide variety of wholesome natural foods.

SUMMARY

To increase your vitamin and mineral intake, augment your diet with special health foods such as brewer's yeast, bone meal, kelp, dolomite, desiccated liver, and Vitamin C tablets.

fifteen

Milk and Egg Machines

Some advocates of nutrition from natural sources are opposed to the use of cow's milk. They remind us that animals drink only the milk of their own species, and that man is the only animal who drinks the milk of another species, such as the cow.

As an additional argument against cow's milk, this school contends that milk is not a natural food for adults, but that it is a growth food, meant only for infants. Man is the only adult animal who drinks milk, for among all other animals, milk is consumed only by the infant. For the human infant, it is recognized that mother's milk is the perfect food. But cow's milk is formulated by nature for the systems of calves, not humans, or so say the anti-milk set.

Why do I advocate cow's milk for adults, when neither ape nor primitive man drank it—nor even drank mother's milk beyond babyhood?

One reason is man's apparent acquired need for animal

97

protein, of which milk is the least putrefactive or toxic.
But another less tangible reason is that since nature designed milk to nourish beginning life, it may also contain
some still-to-be-discovered protective factor. Evidence already exists to the effect that cow's milk contains a yet-
unidentified element that promotes growth. Perhaps it also
contains some protective substance that is advantageous
not only to the calf, but also to the human race, including
adults.

This theory may not be far-fetched. Adele Davis, the
long-experienced and highly regarded nutritionist, states:
"I have yet to know of a single adult developing cancer
who has habitually drunk a quart of milk daily."

Most of the milk sold in this country has been cooked,
or pasteurized. Law requires the pasteurization of milk
because this process kills any potentially harmful germs
that may be present. But while destroying germs, the heat
of pasteurization also destroys some of the food value of
milk. All its enzymes are completely invalidated, and its
vitamins and minerals are damaged. It is estimated that
pasteurization destroys more Vitamin C each year than is
contained in the country's entire citrus crop. As for the
calcium in milk, many nutritionists warn that pasteurization tends to render this important mineral insoluble, and
therefore ineffective for use by the body.

In destroying germs, pasteurization is impartial to both
friend and foe. While killing any unfriendly bacteria that
may be present, it also kills the friendly lactic-acid bacil-
lus, which combats food putrefaction in the intestine.

Boosters of raw food are not in favor of disease germs
in milk, and they concede that raw milk is an ideal
medium for the rapid growth of almost all types of bacteria. Infected milk can, and formerly often did, spread
tuberculosis, typhoid, diphtheria, infant diarrhea, and a
swarm of other diseases.

However, today's sanitary requirements do away with the need for pasteurization, say the raw milk exponents. Dairy barns and equipment are government-inspected regularly for cleanliness and sanitation, the health of dairy cows must meet certain standards, and milk itself must pass bacteriological tests. Milk given the rating of Grade A, claim the raw-milk backers, is safe without pasteurization. In support of their contention that today's clean, raw milk is safe, its advocates offer the following proof.

Before raw milk is picked up by the dairy for pasteurization, some of it is drunk by most dairy farmers and their families. It is also sold "under the counter" directly to consumers who come to the farm by many farmers. No ill effects result; no epidemics occur.

Cynical raw-food advocates allege that the real reason behind pasteurization is the same as that behind other processes which impair natural foods—profit. Among the bacteria killed by pasteurization are the harmless ones that cause milk to sour. Once pasteurized, milk keeps longer, and this enables dairies to distribute milk without spoilage, with a result of greater profit to the dairies.

Those who appreciate the nutritional superiority of raw milk over pasteurized milk suggest an alternative to pasteurization. Raw milk could be preserved from spoiling by keeping it refrigerated at just above the freezing point. Indeed, this is exactly the way today's dairy farmer is required to protect his milk until it is picked up for pasteurization.

If kept at slightly above freezing, raw milk can be stored for weeks, or even months. But keeping milk refrigerated at just above freezing until it reaches the consumer would be more costly and bothersome than pasteurization, so under the guise of protecting the public's health, milk is robbed of some of its health-building qualities.

A form of unpasteurized milk known as "certified raw

milk" may be sold legally in some states. Certified raw milk is produced under strict government control. Cows which produce this milk are fed a carefully balanced diet and are washed and inspected daily. The bacterial count of their milk may not exceed a set limit.

In states where certified raw milk can be sold, it is available only in or near the larger cities. There, the enlightened minority are clustered in sufficient numbers to make production of this superior food profitable. If you don't live where raw milk is available, you can still enjoy many of its benefits, for raw-milk cheese is sold by dairies that advertise in health magazines and by some health-food dealers.

Don't pass up milk or cheese if you can't get them in their raw state, for they still contain much nutritive value even after pasteurization.

Of the many protein foods, eggs are richest in all the essential amino acids. Some nutritionists recommend eating one or more eggs every day. However, other experts advocate a limit of only two or three eggs a week, or even none at all. Although eggs are protein-rich, they are also abundant in artery-clogging cholesterol. By doing without eggs, you'll help keep your arteries clear. But if you do eat eggs, never eat them uncooked. Raw egg white contains an anti-vitamin substance called avidin. Avidin prevents the body from absorbing one of the B Vitamins, biotin. When eggs are cooked, the avidin is deactivated.

In endorsing milk and eggs, many nutritionists do so with some reservation. They decry the artificial conditions under which milk and eggs are produced today.

Normally, a cow gives enough milk for her calf's needs and a little extra. Although the calf takes only a small amount of milk at each feeding, the modern dairy farmer still milks the cow almost dry, which stimulates it to produce more and more milk. Instead of the cow's normal production of about two hundred pounds of milk a year, she is forced to give much more—often as much as twenty thousand or more pounds a year.

No one knows what effect this forced production has on the cow, and in turn on her milk. A reasonable surmise would be that compulsory overproduction of milk lowers its quality.

Eggs, like milk, are also mass-produced now. Just as today's cow is a milk machine, the modern hen has become an egg machine.

Assembly-line eggs were introduced in the 1930's. Before then, chickens were allowed to roam outside—unrestrained, or in a fenced-in yard—where they got the benefits of the outdoors, exercised, and ate a natural diet of seeds, grass, insects, and worms. The hen entered their shelter only when they so desired.

Today's chickens live an unnatural existence. They are born, live out their days, and die indoors, crowded into barracks designed for egg-production. They are fed a diet planned only to make them produce more and more eggs. Lights are kept on for all but a few hours a day, because this stimulates egg-laying. The egg produced under such artificial conditions can only be inferior to the old-fashioned kind.

Another cause of the inferiority of today's eggs is that most of them are laid by hens who never see a rooster. Chickens will lay eggs without there being a rooster in the flock, but such eggs lack the germ of life, and no chick can hatch from them. These sterile eggs are also less nourishing, but they keep better. Why bother with a rooster when chickens will lay just as many eggs without one, and the eggs will keep better?

Eggs produced in the old-fashioned way are sold in

some health-food stores. Here and there, an individual can be found who still keeps chickens the old way on a small scale, and who may be willing to sell some of his flock's output. Watch for a source of natural eggs during short drives in the country. Look for outdoor chickens, either inside a fenced yard or roaming freely.

If the flock is headed by a rooster, all the better. Then you won't have to settle for "old-maid eggs." Instead, you will be eating the output of a rooster-dominated harem of happy hens: eggs that are fertile and natural.

Personally, I have given up eating eggs. Their protein is available from other sources, without the high content of artery-clogging cholesterol.

Summary

If possible, use milk or cheese that is raw, not pasteurized. If possible, use eggs produced by chickens which are allowed outdoors, and from a flock which includes a rooster.

sixteen

The Saturation Diet

Not only the uninitiated run the risk of nutritional shortages in their diet. Even among the health-conscious, food selection is often made on a hit-or-miss basis. Although they eat only wholesome foods, they may make little attempt to insure that they are getting all of the needed elements in sufficient quantities. Many, if not most, of the health-minded don't even know how much of each of the nutrients is needed daily.

Of course, by eating a wide variety of wholesome foods instead of following the average diet, one is sure to come close to getting all the elements he needs. Yet whether all of these elements are present in sufficient quantities is still a gamble. The hit-or-miss eater of health foods may get a plentitude of some elements, yet not enough of others.

How nice it would be if our instincts told us exactly what to eat, and just how much of it, in order to gain the utmost nourishment. It has been said that primitive peoples instinctively select foods containing the elements needed by their bodies, and it has been shown in tests that

young children do the same, provided that they are offered only natural, unrefined foods. However, the rest of
us probably can't depend upon our instincts to guide us in
selecting all the nutrients we need in sufficient quantities.

A better guide to nutrition is provided by the United
States government. Through the Food and Nutrition
Board of the National Research Council, the government
has established the daily minimum requirements for the
various food elements. The recommended allowances are
those considered adequate for good nutrition. The council's tables are used by dietitians as a guide for meal-
planning.

However, a much greater intake than that recommended by the government is urged by some sophisticated
nutritionists. These experts have set their goal higher
than mere freedom from disease. Their purpose is to encourage the utmost in health.

Dr. Henry C. Sherman, who conducted longevity experiments at Columbia University and was recognized as
one of the world's outstanding experts on nutrition,
reached the conclusion that, for optimum nourishment,
vitamins are needed in *four times* the amount generally
recognized as adequate. Dr. Sherman also recommended
two to four times the normal amount of the key mineral
calcium and half again the protein usually considered sufficient. Dr. Sherman's opinions are shared by many modern
nutritionists who believe in supplying the body with every
needed nutrient to the point of saturation.

To keep the body's cells saturated with every necessary
food element would require considerable information on
nutrition, plus very careful meal-planning. But who would
want to have to plan every meal by wading through complicated nutritional charts? Food selection should be fun.
With this in mind, I have prepared a simplified eating
guide that I call the Saturation Diet. Daily intake of the

foods listed in the quantities shown will provide all needed elements in approximately the high quantities recommended by advanced nutritionists like Dr. Sherman.

The three-category Saturation Diet is not a monotonous one. Alternatives are given in some divisions, and foods not listed may be eaten as desired.

THE SATURATION DIET
CATEGORY 1. ANIMAL FOODS (EAT SOME ANIMAL FOOD AT EVERY MEAL):

Milk, or skim milk—1 to 1½ quarts, or 7 to 10 ounces of cheese.

Meat, or fish—1 small serving.

CATEGORY 2. PLANT FOODS (EAT RAW FRUITS AND VEGETABLES IN EVER-CHANGING VARIETIES):

Raw Fruits—several whole fruits, or the equivalent in raw juice.

Raw Vegetables—one large serving of salad containing several different vegetables, or the equivalent in juice.

Raw Nuts, or raw peanuts—one handful.

Raw Sunflower Seeds—one handful.

Oranges—At least six, or 1 pint of orange juice, or several Vitamin C tablets, divided into at least three widely spaced servings.

Raw Carrots, Parsley, Spinach, or Dandelion Greens, or their juice—one large serving.

Legumes, Whole Grains, or Potatoes—As much as desired; govern quantities by checking your weight.

CATEGORY 3. SUPPLEMENTAL FOODS:

Brewer's Yeast—2 heaping teaspoonfuls.

Bone Meal—1 level teaspoonful.

Powdered Kelp—1 level teaspoonful.

Powdered Dolomite—1 level teaspoonful.

Desiccated   Liver   Tablets—Follow   dosage   recommended on container.
Vitamin E Capsules—at least 200 International Units.
Unhydrogenated Vegetable Oil—2 tablespoonfuls.
Sunshine—frequent exposure.

Items are listed in this diet in the amounts needed by adult men. Women and teen-agers require slightly less of some nutrients, but for practical purposes, the guide will also serve them. Pregnant women and nursing mothers require somewhat more of all nutrients. Children's requirements are about half that of adults. Baby feeding should follow your doctor's recommendations and should include raw foods if he permits.

In the Saturation Diet, vegetable protein is derived from nuts or peanuts, brewer's yeast, and sunflower seeds, as well as from some of the other foods.

The need for carbohydrates is fulfilled by the nuts or peanuts, milk, legumes, grain, potatoes, and some of the other foods.

The requirements for unsaturated fats are taken care of by the nuts or peanuts, the sunflower seeds, and by the unhydrogenated vegetable oil, which can be added to a salad.

Vitamins are plentifully present, both in the regular and the supplemental foods. The Vitamin A requirement is fulfilled mainly by the carrots, spinach, or dandelion greens. The entire family of B Vitamins is found both in the brewer's yeast and the desiccated-liver tablets. The frequently needed Vitamin C comes principally from the spaced-out intake of oranges or Vitamin C tablets. Vitamin D is obtained from a non-food source, sunshine. Vitamin E is derived mainly from Vitamin E capsules. (Sufferers from high blood pressure or rheumatic heart disease should take Vitamin E only under the supervision of a doctor.)

The many rich natural sources of calcium, such as raw vegetables, bone meal, and kelp, give you all you need and more of this most important mineral. As for the other minerals, if you get enough calcium from natural sources, you will automatically get enough of the other minerals, which accompany calcium in natural foods.

Supplement potencies are easily calculated. Potency per tablet or per capsule is listed on containers either in milligrams (mg.) or International Units (I. U.). USP is the equivalent of I. U.

A microgram (mcg.) is the equivalent of 1/1000 of a milligram.

This section on nutrition has been lengthy because it is the subject on which the most material is available. Among health scholars, nutrition has been ranked higher in importance, and has been given far more study, than have the other factors affecting health and longevity.

Though I rate two other factors above nutrition (we'll discuss them later), I do not mean to underestimate the significance of proper diet. The right diet has contributed enormously to keeping the seven girls and two boys in our family in excellent health, so I'm not deprecating the nutritionists. I owe them too much.

SUMMARY

To keep your cells saturated with every needed food element, follow the Saturation Diet daily.

seventeen

Too Few Chew

Back in 1893, at the age of forty-four, Horace Fletcher applied for a life-insurance policy and was rejected. Reading the handwriting on the wall, Fletcher also began to read something else: books on health. From his studies, he developed a health and longevity idea which he subsequently publicized as a panacea for man's ills.

According to Fletcher, nature placed teeth in the mouth for a reason. He concluded that each mouthful of food should be chewed until it turned to a semiliquid. Only then was it fit to be swallowed.

Books on the new discovery, written not only by Fletcher but also by his disciples, spread this message. *Cosmopolitan*, the *Ladies' Home Journal*, *McClure's*, and other popular magazines of the day also heralded this message. By 1909, more than two hundred thousand American families were "Fletcherizing" three times a day, and chewing their way to health.

Today Fletcherizing has been forgotten by all but a few "faddists." In fact, this subject is scarcely mentioned today, except for laughs. But in this age of eat-and-run, the time has perhaps come to stop treating Fletcherizing as a joke and to revive the healthful practice of chewing.

Too few people chew their food thoroughly enough. I suggest that you try a little experiment the next time you eat. Chew a mouthful of food in the same way you always do, but check yourself when you are at the point of swallowing. Instead of swallowing, feel the food with your tongue. You will probably be surprised to find poorly chewed lumps in the food that you were about to swallow.

There are two good reasons for thoroughly chewing your food: (1) The nourishment in food is locked in its cells. Unless these cells are broken down, many nutrients remain locked in, and (2) Chewing causes the digestive juices in the mouth to mix with the food.

Proteins, carbohydrates, and fats can all be digested more efficiently if they are chewed well.

Proteins are converted into usable amino acids in your stomach. Even if you don't bother to chew steak thoroughly, your stomach will manage to digest it after a fashion, but it will need to work harder. To do the job, it will have to secrete more hydrochloric acid—up to three or four times as much as if your teeth had done more of the work.

Even more important than thorough chewing of proteins is thorough chewing of carbohydrates. The digestion of these begins in the mouth, where they mix with certain enzymes to begin the chemical process of digestion.

Plenty of chewing is also highly important during a meal which contains fat. Fat doesn't start to digest until it reaches the intestines. In the meantime, on the way to the intestines, fat hinders the digestion of other foods. In the mouth, fat covers carbohydrates and hinders penetration by the digestive juices. In the stomach, fat covers the proteins and inhibits digestion. But if foods containing fat are chewed well, the digestive juices can reach the proteins and carbohydrates more easily.

In addition to the nutritional rewards, chewing your food well brings you another benefit. Your teeth were meant to be used, and exercising makes them stronger and healthier and lessens your chances of dental trouble.

But better nutrition and sounder teeth aren't the only advantages to be gained by developing the habit of thorough mastication. In addition, the chewing habit, once learned, adds greatly to mealtime enjoyment. Why not prolong and intensify this enjoyment? Why rush tasty morsels down? Once the habit of thorough chewing has become firmly fixed, eating will become more enjoyable.

Learning the chewing habit requires a little practice. At first, it must be done consciously. But the habit is quickly learned, and it will soon become automatic. The three rules for slower chewing and more food enjoyment are: (1) Take smaller mouthfuls, (2) Chew at a slower rate, and (3) Chew each mouthful longer.

If these rules are followed consciously, especially at the beginning of each meal, the habit of chewing thoroughly will soon be learned.

If lack of teeth prevents your chewing certain hard foods, this job can be turned over to a machine. Health-food dealers sell a small electrical appliance made expressly for grinding hard foods. Seeds, nuts, and other hard-to-chew foods are quickly ground to a soft pulp by this device.

This ground pulp could be swallowed almost without chewing, but you should still go through the motions of thorough chewing in order to mix the food thoroughly with saliva. For the same reason, all liquids except water should be chewed just like solid foods. Milk and juices contain natural sugars, the digestion of which must begin in the mouth. Each mouthful should be masticated in the same way as solid food, or if you prefer, you can imitate the nursing infant, and chew your liquids by taking little tiny sips, which automatically mix with the digestive juices.

One reason cooked food is popular is that it is easier to chew. Cooking softens food, and this makes eating easier —too much easier. Soft food can be gulped down with very little mastication.

Cooking substitutes for chewing in still another way. The heat of cooking releases nutrients from food cells by breaking down the tough, fibrous cell walls. At the same time, of course, the heat damages the very vitamins and minerals it releases, and it also kills the enzymes.

SUMMARY

To chew your food thoroughly, take smaller mouthfuls, chew at a slower rate, and chew each mouthful longer.

eighteen

The Mini-Menu

Eat less. This is another secret of good health and long life. The undereater is healthier than the overeater. The undereater doesn't burden his body with excessive food-handling chores, nor with excess weight.

The first rule for the moderate eater is to always stop eating while you are still a little hungry. If you always leave the table feeling that you could have eaten a little more, your digestive and assimilative apparatus will have it easier.

Another way to undertax your system is to avoid eating between meals. If you eat only at mealtime, your stomach has time to digest each meal and then rest a while before the next meal. But if you indulge in between-meal snacks, even little ones, your food-handling machinery is working more than it should be.

The disadvantages of between-meal eating are seldom stressed, or even mentioned, by those who write on nutrition, but I feel that eating only at mealtime is an important health rule.

Thirty-eight years ago when my interest in the pursuit

of good health was born, one of the first dietary rules I began to observe was not eating between meals. At that time,
my former headaches stopped. I have stuck with this rule,
and my headaches have never returned. In fact, I have
forgotten exactly how a headache feels. I don't know
whether or not between-meal eating is related to headaches, but there is some evidence that this may be so. If
you suffer from headaches, you have possibly just learned
how to find relief.

We Prohaskas all follow the "nothing-between-meals"
rule. This keeps the children's appetites sharp. Unlike
children who nibble during the day and then aren't hungry at mealtime, the young Prohaskas bring good appetites to the table. They do not need to be coaxed into eating the healthful food set before them.

Whenever you feel the need for a between-meal snack,
eat raw fruit or drink unsweetened fruit juice. This
quickly digested and nutritious food should satisfy your
craving, and it won't overtax your digestive system.

Another rule for the undereater is to eat only when hungry. If you aren't hungry, when mealtime arrives, don't
eat.

Most people are horrified at the thought of skipping a
meal, but it does no harm whatever to miss an occasional
meal. On the contrary, it can do much good. Your physical
system will get a needed rest—the rest it was asking for by
signaling that it was not hungry. Chances are that when
mealtime comes around again, your appetite will have returned. This will be another kind of signal from your body
—a sign that it is now ready for food.

What about healthy oldsters? Do their feeding habits
support the theory that moderate eating is conducive to
better health and longer life?

For the most part, the healthy and long-lived are undereaters. More than three-quarters of those in the Gallup survey have been careful not to eat too much all their lives. They either seldom or never ate bedtime snacks. Less than one-fourth of them ate between meals. Rarely, reports Dr. Gallup, have any of these oldsters been fat.

In the land of the Hunzans, food, though nutritious, is scarce. Although no one starves, there just isn't enough food to permit anyone to overeat. The Hunzan food allowance is rated by one observer as "practically a starvation diet."

Like the Hunzans, the long-lived Russian peasants have to wrest their food from the soil, and, being subject to the vagaries of weather, their crops are not always abundant. In discussing a study of Russians over one hundred years of age, *Geriatrics* magazine says: "The people who have reached such a ripe old age by no means led a shielded life. On the contrary, most of them experienced many hardships, and there were times when they did not eat sufficiently." [1]

To help your body work better and last longer, join the undereaters.

SUMMARY

Always stop eating while still a little hungry, and never eat anything except raw fruit or raw fruit juice between meals. Moreover, eat only when hungry, even if this means skipping an occasional meal.

[1] *Geriatrics*, July, 1965.

nineteen

The Pushers

A new hazard to health and longevity has developed recently, one which scarcely existed in 1900. Even in the 1930's when I first became health-conscious, this hazard was only minor. Today, it has become a major peril to health and longevity. This new danger is chemical poisoning.

Although you may not be aware of it, poison enters your body from many sources in frequent daily doses. We are living in the age of chemicals. Our food is heavily treated with chemicals in various ways by the farmer who grows it. Four hundred thousand tons of pest-killing chemicals alone are used each year. Moreover, many foods are colored, flavored, and preserved by means of the addition of various chemicals—3,700 different ones. In addition, the air we breathe is severely polluted by industry, automobile exhausts, and other offenders. For example, motor vehicles each year eject into the air more than ninety million tons of chemicals.

Still other sources add to this chemical cloudburst. Cigarette smokers inhale poison with every puff. Drinkers partake of a well-known poisonous chemical, alcohol. Those who take medicines add to their chemical intake. Every dose of medicine is also a dose of poison. Pain-killers, tranquilizers, and other such remedies are all compounded of chemicals.

Miscellaneous other sources add still more to this deluge. Frequent doses of poison come from all sides.

This constant barrage of chemicals leads to the accumulation of poisons in the body. This poison build-up, according to experts who have investigated the problem, may eventually lead to disease. Many sicknesses may actually be cases of delayed poisoning in disguise.

Some authorities place much of the blame for today's growing increase in cancer on chemical pollution. One expert who connects cancer with the age of poison is Dr. Philippe Shubik, director of the Eppley Institute for Cancer Research at the University of Nebraska. Says Dr. Shubik: "Within the past decade particularly, it has become apparent that chemical carcinogenic factors may well be responsible for a large number of cancers in man. An expert committee for the World Health Organization, writing on cancer, concluded that at least 50% of all cancers in human beings could be considered to be caused by extrinsic environmental agents." [1]

Despite expert opinion that environmental chemicals are linked to the incidence of cancer in man, chemical companies continue to pollute human bodies. Justifying their contaminants is easy. Many poisons contribute to, or are the result of, some useful economic function. Compared to the benefits they offer, the accompanying harm to human health is claimed to be negligible. When no ex-

[1] *National Tattler*, August 10, 1969.

cuse can be found for a poison, as with cigarettes or alcohol, the resulting harm is either blamed on other causes or minimized.

A favorite dodge of the chemical dispensers and their publicists is that poisons are being restricted to "safe" levels. The small dosages in which poisons enter the human body are dismissed as being harmless. But those who have become alarmed at this chemicalization point out that the effects of a poison may be cumulative. Many small, harmless doses can add up to one large, harmful dose.

Dramatic proof of poison's cumulative effect on the body emerged only a few years ago. This new evidence should have put a stop to the claims that repeated small doses of poison are harmless, for the very opposite was demonstrated in 1964 by Surgeon-General Terry's report which connected lung cancer and other serious ailments with cigarette-smoking. Lung cancer is never brought on by smoking a single cigarette, or even a few. The smoker develops the disease only after many years of smoking, yet, the lung-cancer victim smoked only one "harmless" cigarette at a time.

DDT is another poison whose long-term dangerous effects have finally been recognized. When DDT was introduced in the early 1940's, it was hailed as a miracle-worker. Its use in the prevention of insect-borne diseases saved countless lives overseas.

Then, farmers in this country adopted it to keep their crops free of insects because it was cheap and easy to use. Concerned observers warned that this insect-killer would eventually kill people, for it is impossible to remove by ordinary means the residue of this poison which remains on the surfaces of sprayed foods. In addition, more poison is absorbed as the plant feeds. Along with food, consumers were imbibing deadly poison.

Warnings against this were pooh-poohed by propagandists for the chemical industry. As late as 1968, an author who had been brainwashed by these chemists wrote: "Human beings seem able to take aboard quite large amounts of DDT without apparent harm." (This same statement could have been made about cigarette smoke only a few years previously.)

Despite more and more proof of the accumulation of DDT in the body tissue of Americans, the government permitted the increasing use of this pesticide. Finally, late in 1969, nearly thirty years after the introduction of DDT, its health-destroying potential was officially recognized, and the government acted to outlaw DDT for all but essential uses.

In the meantime, this poison has been doing its dirty work in two hundred million American bodies. This persistent pesticide is found not only in most foodstuffs, but also in samples of body fat selected from people at random, in mother's milk, and in the cells of unborn children.

And despite the fact that DDT's villainy has at last been acknowledged, the use of this poison has only been reduced, not forbidden. In 1970, the year after DDT was outlawed, the United States chemical industry still produced this potent pollutant at the rate of seventy thousand tons annually.

Another type of offender, which has long been officially considered innocent even after being proven guilty, is cyclamates, the artificial sweeteners.

Cyclamates became suspect soon after their introduction, when research began to uncover evidence of their ill effects on the body. The Wisconsin Alumni Research Foundation proved, in tests on animals, that cyclamates brought on various ill effects, including mental retardation and retarded growth. At the University of Washington in Seattle, cyclamates were found to affect blood pressure and heartbeat. Still other research piled up more and more evidence against these chemical sweeteners, but the laboratories not only continued to make cyclamates, they also issued statements that whitewashed their ill effects.

The government suddenly ordered cyclamates off the market nearly twenty years after their introduction. In the meantime, the consumption of cyclamates had reached fifteen million pounds a year. These chemicals had been used to sweeten more than seven hundred products, including aspirin and vitamins made especially for children.

The dangers to the human body of the three poisons just discussed have now been recognized, and something more or less is belatedly being done about them. But what about all the other chemicals to which we are exposed which are still officially considered safe? How many of these will future research prove capable of causing harm to the human body in varying degrees?

And what about the *new* poisons that are currently being developed? How many of them will be rushed into production and distribution without regard for the safety of consumers?

SUMMARY

Chemical poisoning from many sources is a relatively recent hazard to health and long life to which people are exposed today.

twenty

Invisible Invaders

For two million years, man lived in a clean, chemical-free world. Today, he suddenly finds himself surrounded by poisons. His body must try to cope with hundreds, even thousands, of foreign substances which were never meant to enter the human body. The following is a closer look at some of the poisons by which today's American is assaulted.

Today, crops are grown with the help of chemicals, for growing food is subject to insect damage, and damaged crops mean less profit. Therefore, fruits and vegetables are protected from insects by poisonous pesticide sprays. But some of the poison meant for the insects remains on the plants, impervious to ordinary washing, and some of it soaks into the ground, to be absorbed as the plant feeds. In this way, some of the poisonous pesticide ends up on the inside of the consumer's body.

Moreover, the animals on most farms are also given chemical treatment. These animals are dosed with hormones, antibiotics, tranquilizers, and other drugs which promote greater and faster growth and prevent or treat disease. Traces of these chemicals may remain in the meat, milk, or eggs that we eat.

Stilbestrol, a hormone, is one commonly used chemical. An article in *Successful Farming* magazine urges farmers to administer this drug to their beef cattle. This article promises that if stilbestrol is fed to or implanted in an animal, it will promote a weight gain of from thirty-five to fifty pounds. "In terms of dollars and cents, this is $8–$12 more per animal. Cost of stilbestrol—about 35¢." But the ultimate cost of stilbestrol to the secondhand consumer could be much higher. William Longgood writes, in his book *The Poisons in Your Food:* "The substance is an acknowledged carcinogen, and warnings against its use have been sounded by Dr. Heuper and the International Union Against Cancer."

The farmer's chemicalized vegetables, fruits, and livestock may win blue ribbons at the county fair, but they can be the cause of your losing your health.

Moreover, the pollution of food doesn't stop with the farmer. Between the farmer and the consumer stands the fellow who processes and packages food. Under the guise of improving food by making it look, taste, smell, or keep better, the processor is able to make it sell better.

Acidifiers and alkalizers, bleaches and buffers, dyes and deodorants, emulsifiers and extenders, flavorers and fortifiers, stabilizers and sweeteners, thinners and thickeners, and many other chemical creations are added to your food, and thus enter your body.

In 1959, an estimated four hundred chemicals were being added to foods. Only nine years later, in 1968, this figure had shot up to two thousand four hundred and by now the chemical industry has undoubtedly come up with many new food pollutants. Understandably, chemical manufacturers encourage chemicalization. Like farmers and food processors, chemical makers aren't in business for their health, nor for yours!

Pharmaceutical companies are among the leading producers of chemicals for human consumption. Annual sales of prescription medicines total over three billion dollars. The sale of tranquilizers alone amounts to four hundred and twelve million dollars a year. Of non-prescription pills, aspirin, just one, accounts for annual sales of over four hundred and eighty-three million dollars. (Americans take twenty-seven *tons* of aspirin a *day!*)

Those who seek health from the drugstore may get just the opposite. Every dose of medicine is a potential dose of poison. Pain-killers, tranquilizers, sedatives, antibiotics, and other medicines are godsends if and when they are really needed. But they are also poisonous chemicals. They accomplish their good works by altering natural bodily functions, and as chemicals, they are capable of harmful as well as beneficial action.

Proof of harmful reactions to drugs is sometimes quick in coming, for the administration of a drug sometimes causes skin rash, nausea, vomiting, diarrhea, or other such symptoms. Sometimes, these reactions take a more serious form and result in damage to internal organs, and occasionally death.

Anyone who doubts that drugs can cause harmful effects should read the advertisements in medical journals. These ads, placed by drug manufacturers, are directed to doctors, and while promoting a specific drug, they also warn of harmful side effects that have been observed in connection with the use of a particular drug. An advertisement for a pain reliever in *Archives of Surgery* devoted twenty-two lines of small type to a cataloguing of its possible side effects, among which were nausea, vomiting, constipation, irritability, and headache.

A more sinister warning stated that when a particular drug was used in large amounts or for long periods of time, it might cause kidney damage.

In an ad for a tranquilizer which appeared in *Medical Economics*, twenty lines of fine print were needed to discuss its possible harmful side effects, among which were dizziness, headache, skin rash, gastrointestinal disturbances, and fever. This advertisement also mentioned some more-serious consequences, including two fatalities.

Side Effects of Drugs, a medical book, has over five hundred pages devoted to the description of the harmful effects of drugs as they have been observed by doctors.

But the side effects listed in drug ads and medical books are usually only the immediate and more-obvious ones. Drug reactions are sometimes delayed. When they finally occur, they may be blamed on something other than the drug that was the responsible or contributing factor.

Use of one or more so-called harmless medicines over a period of time, especially when coupled with routine ingestion of various other poisons, may ultimately cause serious disease. One such possible result that has been mentioned by many is cancer.

Pat McGrady, a medical writer who suggests the possible link between medical drugs and cancer, says: "One question that haunts the researcher who studies the behavior of cancer is this: Can it sometimes be caused by the drugs prescribed to fight disease or by the doctor treating the patient?" [1] Mr. McGrady goes on to discuss the group of drugs known as phenols. Regarding these commonly used drugs, McGrady writes: "University of Wis-

[1] Albany, New York, *Times-Union*, April 17, 1965.

consin scientists, testing more than fifty phenols, found that over half caused animal cancers, and they concluded 'the hazards to man must now be considered.' "

Although drugs save countless lives, they are also capable of *taking* lives. Many uneasy observers, some of whom are doctors, feel that drugs are being overused.

Unlike other poisoners, air polluters do not deliberately produce poisons, but produce them as by-products.

The sources of air pollution are many, including automobile exhausts, industrial processes, burning of heating fuels, municipal garbage incineration, and burning of refuse.

How serious is the effect of air pollution on the human body? Dr. Stephen Ayres, chest specialist at St. Vincent's Hospital in New York City, says: "There is little doubt that living in a polluted area is like taking a few years off your life."

The life-shortening effects of air pollution have been detailed in many studies which compared residents of heavily polluted areas with residents of less-polluted regions nearby. For example, one such survey, headed by Dr. Warren Winklestein of the University of Buffalo School of Medicine, involved men between the ages of fifty and sixty-nine, who were on the same economic level. Those living in the least-polluted section of Buffalo were compared with those living in the most-polluted part. Deaths from all causes in the polluted area were one-third higher than those in the less-polluted area.

The automobile is the leading air polluter. Analysis of automobile-exhaust gases reveals that they contain more than two hundred different chemicals. Let us consider lead; just one of these potential health-destroying poisons. I have done some extra study of this pollutant for a personal reason—my proneness to gout. Mention that you are subject to attacks of gout, and you often get a knowing smile, for gout is popularly associated with the heavy consumption of rich foods and alcoholic beverages. In truth, the basic cause of gout is an inherited metabolic defect. (More than one hundred such inheritable defects are known.) Those subject to gout may contract it, even if they do not overindulge. Despite my health program, I have suffered many painful bouts of gout.

Lead in the human system is a contributing cause of gout—a fact which has been known for over two hundred years. In former days, when lead was an ingredient of most house paints, gout was a common ailment of house painters. Today, doctors are puzzled over the rising incidence of this malady. I think I can show them one reason for this.

Our environment has become heavily contaminated with lead from various sources, but mainly from automobile exhausts. An article in *New Yorker* magazine states: "Our supplies of food and water contain twenty times as much lead as they did in primitive days." This increase in environmental lead content can be verified. One way to do so is to check old trees. Study of the rings in these trees reveals that the newest rings contain twenty-four times as much lead as rings that are one hundred years old.

Further evidence of increasing lead in the environment comes from testing deep layers of snow. *Fortune* magazine states: "A Caltech geochemist, Clair C. Patterson, reported increased amounts of lead in the upper layers of snows in the high Rockies and in Greenland over those in the deeper snows of yesteryear, from which he calculated that people are now carrying one hundred times more lead than they once did." [2] *Time* magazine indicates that the human lead burden is even higher: "In the auto's

2 *Fortune*, July, 1967.

70-year history, the average American's lead content has risen an estimated 125-fold, to near maximum tolerance levels."

Today, almost all gasoline is leaded. Car exhausts discharge this lead into the air we breathe. In London, the air in the middle of a busy street was found to contain four times the lead of the air in less-traveled areas. In the United States, an estimated two hundred million pounds of lead are spewed from auto-exhaust pipes annually—nearly one pound for every inhabitant.

Still more lead enters human systems at second hand. Crops grown near busy roads absorb some atmospheric lead. Vegetables picked within twenty-five feet of roads were found to contain four times as much lead as those grown five hundred feet away.

In addition to the lead from car exhausts, other sources that add to lead bombardment are some insecticides, cigarette smoke, and fumes and dust from certain industrial plants.

Just how dangerous is this poisonous substance which is now so prevalent in our environment and in our bodies?

The American Conference of Governmental Industrial Hygienists has adopted threshold-limit values for industrial atmospheric contaminants. Although the organization's recommendations are intended for evaluation of industrial rather than community air-pollution problems, their findings are highly revealing. While the threshold limits permitted for some contaminants run as high as one thousand parts per million parts of air, the tolerance limit for lead is zero.

What are the likely consequences to health when lead enters the human body? According to *Fortune* magazine: ". . . lead . . . once it gets inside the human body in any sizable quantity, is a highly toxic substance, tending to impair the functioning of the blood, kidneys, liver, and central nervous system." [3]

The lead in our environment is undoubtedly affecting not only health but also life itself. In experiments on rats in which the animals were given lead in the approximate quantities present in our environment, 57% of the rats died within twenty-three months. At the same time, in rats kept free from lead, the death rate was only 10%.

This brings me back to the subject of gout. Unless you are already predisposed to the ailment, an excess of lead finding its way into your system will probably fail to bring on gout. But who knows what other harm lead may be doing inside your body? In addition, lead is only one of the over two hundred chemicals ejected from car exhausts. If lead doesn't do you in, perhaps one of the other chemicals will.

How much does smoking and drinking contribute to a person's cumulative total of poison? Plenty, as is proved by statistics. According to the Public Health Service, the average man who continues to be a heavy cigarette-smoker throughout his life will die eight years sooner than the non-smoker.

Heavy drinking is an even greater life-shortener than heavy smoking. Dr. Andrew C. Ivy of the University of Illinois has provided an astounding statistic: The average life span of the alcoholic is nineteen years less than that of the non-alcoholic.

Miscellaneous other poisons add their bit to the terrible total.

Coffee and tea, even when unsugared, contain harmful substances.

[3] *Fortune,* July, 1967.

Although almost everyone is aware that coffee contains caffeine, it is not commonly known that considerable caffeine is also present in cola drinks, chocolate, and tea. (Tea also contains two other harmful substances, tannic acid and phylline.) Caffeine is a deadly poison. One drop of caffeine injected into an animal will kill it almost instantly.

The reason one cup of coffee or a glass of cola doesn't kill you is that the caffeine in them is diluted, and most of it is quickly excreted by the kidneys. But even though the drink that contains caffeine doesn't kill you (not immediately, anyway), some of the things it does do immediately are: (1) increases your heartbeat by 15%, (2) increases your respiration by 13%, (3) increases your metabolism rate by up to 25%, (4) increases your stomach's secretion of hydrochloric acid by up to 400%, and (5) narrows the blood vessels in your brain.

Although caffeine is not as potent as some other stimulants, it is a drug, and like many drugs, caffeine is habit-forming. The caffeine in coffee beans, tea leaves, and cola nuts gives coffee, tea, and cola sellers an advantage in the competition for the consumers' beverage dollar.

Not even our drinking water is free from poison. Municipal water departments commonly add twenty-five or more chemicals to water for various reasons, such as to kill bacteria, to control invisible water plants, or to improve the taste.

No one would deny that all these chemicals are added to our drinking water for good reasons. But after they have done their good work, at least traces of them remain to pollute the body of the drinker. Copper sulphate, the chemical most often used to control certain water algae, can also aid in the formation of dangerous fatty deposits on artery walls. Chlorine kills not only the harmful bacteria in the intestinal tract, but also the beneficial kind.

Fluorides which help prevent tooth decay can also inter-fere with the body's absorption of calcium.

Until very recently, when the health dangers of pollu-tion finally began to get a long-overdue airing, few people were even aware that they were being poisoned by pesti-cide residues, food additives, and polluted air.

Meanwhile, many other common poisons are not gener-ally even considered harmful. My generation is aghast at the young people today who poison themselves with nar-cotics. Yet, the overwhelming majority of my generation is hooked on a multitude of more or less potent drugs which are habit-forming in varying degrees. However, we don't call them drugs. We dignify them with names like cigarettes, alcohol, cola drinks, coffee, sugar, tranquilizers, or pep pills. Regardless of the aliases by which we know them, we still become addicted to their poisons, allow them to damage our health, and very often even die of them.

SUMMARY

The main sources of the harmful poisons which find their way into human bodies are farm insecticides and farm-animal drugs, food additives, medicine, air pollution, cigarette-smoking, alcoholic beverages, coffee and tea, and municipal drinking water.

twenty-one

Avoiding the Assassins

Living in a poisoned world as you do, how can you avoid the chemicals that are attacking you from all sides? How can you keep from committing slow suicide?

There are two avenues of escape: Avoid whatever poisons you can, and neutralize, as much as possible, the effects of those poisons you can't avoid.

One way to cut down on poison intake is to select as much of your diet as is practical from among those foods which are least subject to pesticide poisoning. In this category are fruits and vegetables with thick, inedible outer coverings and vegetables that grow underground.

Among the foods that are packaged by nature in throwaway covers which protect them against contamination from direct sprays are nuts, peanuts, peas, beans (including soybeans), corn, bananas, avocados, melons, pumpkins, squash, oranges, grapefruit, tangerines, and pineapples. Among the underground vegetables protected from direct spraying (although they may still absorb some poisons from the soil) are potatoes, carrots, beets, turnips, radishes, and similar vegetables.

The fruits that are most likely to be heavily sprayed, and whose consumption therefore is best avoided or curtailed, are apples, pears, plums, and grapes, with apples probably being the most heavily sprayed of all.

Vegetables to go easy on are the leafy kind, such as lettuce, celery, cabbage, and other greens. These leafy vegetables are important to the diet, but they are most subject to insect attack and therefore are sprayed most heavily. Some authorities advise you to discard the outer leaves of cabbage and head lettuce.

Thin-skinned fruits and leafy vegetables are protective foods that should be eaten regularly; yet these products are the ones most heavily sprayed. Is there a way to include these necessary foods in your diet and still avoid the poisons used in growing them? A partial solution is to clean these foods with a special solvent, a chemical which removes chemicals, that can be obtained from health-food dealers. According to the label on one such product, the material completely removes DDT from the exterior of fruits and vegetables. It should, therefore, have a strong effect on other chemicals too. This method won't get at the poisons a plant may have absorbed, but it will at least remove any residue that remains on the surface.

If you wish, you can easily make your own pesticide remover. The formula is a simple one, with only a single ingredient plus water.

Buy a solution of 10% dilute hydrochloric acid from your drugstore. Mix eight tablespoons of this solution with one gallon of water. Soak fruits and vegetables in this solution for half an hour to remove pesticide residue, then rinse thoroughly in cold running water.

Nature protects seed foods against poisons. These foods

possess a natural ability to repel poisonous chemicals. Which are the seed foods? All nuts, including peanuts, are seeds. So are peas, beans, and corn. Also in this category are specialties sold by health-food dealers, such as sunflower, pumpkin, and sesame seeds.

Farm chemicals can be avoided entirely by eating products that have been raised without chemicals. Such organic foods are available to those who seek to avoid poisoned produce. A growing awareness of the food-pollution problem has created a demand for unchemicalized organic foods. This new market for organically raised products is catered to by a few progressive (or should they be called "old-fashioned"?) farmers. Organic crops are grown in naturally fertilized, rather than chemically fertilized, soils and are never treated with insecticides.

If you are lucky, there may be a farmer near you who does not believe in chemicals and who will sell you his produce. Inquiries among farmers in your vicinity may reveal one or more who grow crops the old way.

Organically raised foods are also available at health-food stores, or they can be ordered by mail from organic farmers and dealers who advertise in health magazines. We Prohaskas buy some of our groceries from organic farms that are several hundred miles away.

Advertisements of organic-food growers and shippers appear regularly in these magazines:

Prevention, Rodale Press, Inc., Emmaus, Pennsylvania 18049

Organic Gardening, Rodale Press, Inc., Emmaus, Pennsylvania 18049

Natural Food and Farming, Natural Food Associates, Inc., P.O. Box 210, Atlanta, Texas 75551. Organically grown foods cost a little more, but they are worth *much* more than they cost.

Another way to avoid food poisons is to raise your own food supply (or at least part of it), using the organic method. A back yard garden can provide a family with a large part of the vegetables it needs. A few fruit trees can furnish healthful desserts.

If you have insufficient space, or can spare but little time for organic gardening, you would be wise to concentrate on raising greens, for you can avoid the most heavily sprayed class of produce on the commercial market by raising your own greens. Not much space is needed to grow greens, and even a small plot can provide the family with a plentiful supply.

Thousands of health-minded people now grow part of their food supply, using the organic system of gardening. Plenty of literature is available to help them grow crops by using this method. This subject is dealt with in both *Organic Gardening* and *Natural Food and Farming* magazines. These publications also carry advertisements for books on organic gardening and farming.

Still another way to avoid food chemicals is to obtain part of your food from plants that grow wild. Apples, dandelion greens, berries, and many other excellent foods can often be found growing wild.

Now what about animal products? These too are subject to pollution from poison. How can you secure unpoisoned animal protein?

Meat from animals raised without chemical contamination is sold by only a few organic farmers, but one kind of nourishing and usually poison-free animal protein is readily available. Fresh ocean fish, rich in protein and minerals, are usually untainted by chemicals. Despite the fact that the ocean is the eventual dumping ground for many chemical poisons, these substances are diluted enough to insure that most ocean fish are poison-free.

Fish is richer in protein than meat, and it has the added

advantage of being cheaper. Consequently, one is sensible to depend more on ocean fish for animal protein than on meat.

Don't use fish from inland waterways, for such fish are often heavily polluted, and don't eat shellfish of any kind, because these fish live near the mouths of rivers, which are also often badly polluted.

In addition to being better for your health, organic foods also have better flavor. Those who sample organically raised foods often express surprise at their superior flavor. If you are old enough to remember how foods used to taste before modern methods of farming came into use, the taste of certain organic foods will bring back memories. Chicken, for example, once possessed a distinctive flavor, but modern battery-raised hens taste bland. Once when we were on vacation in the country, we bought a couple of chickens at a nearby grocery. The birds must have been raised in the old-fashioned outdoor way, because they had that wonderful old-time flavor.

Other foods that now taste different to me than they did when I was young are potatoes, eggs, and grapes.

Anyone who has tasted certain untreated foods that grow wild knows that their flavor is far superior to that of the cultured variety. Cultivated strawberries, for instance, though far larger, are no flavor match for wild strawberries.

What about all the chemicals that have been added to color, flavor, preserve, and otherwise treat the foods that you buy? How can you avoid the harmful additives in food products that have been prettily packaged by their processors?

Some authorities on healthful eating bluntly advise against buying anything that has been packaged. Packaging is usually just the final step the processor takes in tampering with food. This rule doesn't hold good for poison-free packaged foods obtained from a health-food dealer. However, for reasons like economy or convenience, you may wish to get some of your food supply from a supermarket. How can you protect yourself to at least some extent from the many chemical additives in packaged foods? Become a label-reader.

Federal law requires that a listing of all the ingredients, good and bad, appear on most packaged foods. This fine print on the labels often gives away many of the processor's secrets.

There are some exceptions. Congress has exempted certain "standardized" products from these labeling requirements. Mayonnaise, ice cream, and processed cheese are some of the foods which you must purchase without being able to check the ingredients. You would be wise to pass up any packaged foods that do not carry a listing of their ingredients.

Packaged foods, such as raisins or dried beans, carry no such listings. However, these single-ingredient products are obviously unsullied by added chemicals.

If you haven't been checking labels up to now, you are in for some interesting reading. I find it interesting to study food labels in supermarkets, even though most of the packages I check end up back on the shelf. Among the reasons for this are these additives: monosodium glutamate, sulphur dioxide, BHT, BHA, diglycerides, benzoate of soda, alum, sodium propionate, tri-calcium phosphate, and those almost unavoidable poisons, sugar and salt.

Despite the poisons in the packages, I don't return from my supermarket treasure hunts empty-handed. I choose those packaged foods that have been least-abused by the processors. Some of the special gems I have found are corn chips made of whole-grain corn (stone-ground, besides), bread made from stone-ground whole wheat,

and peanut butter without *any* additives (not even hydrogenated oil).

Air pollution is the poisoning it is hardest to avoid.
If you live in or near an industrial area or near a heavily
traveled road, you can't avoid inhaling life-shortening
chemicals. In such cases, your only solution is to move
to a relatively unpolluted area, if circumstances will permit this. Otherwise, you can get cleaner air at least part
of the time by visiting the country on weekends, holidays,
and whenever else it is possible.

One kind of polluted air you *can* keep out of your lungs
is cigarette smoke. Although the best time to stop smoking is before you start, it is never too late to quit. Ex-
smokers live longer than those who continue to smoke.

Evidence seems to indicate that cigar and pipe smoking are far less harmful to the health than cigarette smoking. The reason most commonly given is that cigar and
pipe smokers don't inhale. If you find it impossible to
stop smoking, why not switch to cigars or a pipe?

Women smokers and male smokers who inhale should
switch to cigars or pipes. One young lady I know smokes
cigarettes in public, but in the privacy of her room she
smokes a pipe. But I have seen women smoking cigars in
public, and surprisingly enough, no one pays much attention. If more women smoked cigars or pipes in public, it
would probably soon become acceptable.

Now that I have told you how to smoke in relative
safety, I will tell you how to drink without danger.

Although I have never developed the smoking habit,
I did develop a desire for a nightly bottle of beer. But
after years of drinking and feeling guilty, I finally gave
this up.

For many years thereafter, I took a drink only on special occasions. But one day while I was doing some research in a medical library, I was amazed to find convincing evidence that a light consumption of alcohol is not only harmless, but is actually considered somewhat beneficial.

The evidence in favor of light drinking that I found was compiled by Dr. Raymond Pearl, the researcher who has done so much other work in the field of longevity. Dr. Pearl conducted post-mortem checks of the drinking habits of over five thousand people. He separated them into three categories: nondrinkers, light drinkers, and heavy drinkers. As could be expected, he found that heavy drinkers died much younger than light drinkers or teetotalers. But surprisingly, he also found that *light* drinkers lived slightly longer than *nondrinkers*.

Because Dr. Pearl's findings contradicted the accepted viewpoint and I had read much that supported this viewpoint, I looked for flaws in his evidence. I pondered the possibility that some unsuspected human element might have influenced his statistics. But apparently, this isn't so. Dr. Pearl's findings concerning the effects of light drinking on human life span have been tested in experiments with animals. In repeated tests on dogs, rabbits, and rats, those animals which were regularly given small portions of alcohol lived longer than the teetotaling animals.

Then what about all the studies that had supposedly proved the dire effects of drinking on health and longevity? Actually, these studies only compared teetotalers with *heavy* drinkers. Dr. Pearl also did this, but in addition, he compared teetotalers and *light* drinkers. He thus proved that it is not drinking that shortens life, but *heavy* drinking.

Despite opinion to the contrary—even among many drinkers—and despite all the anti-alcohol propaganda, no conclusive proof exists that moderate drinking is harmful in the least.

John Tobe, the health-book author, concedes, ". . . I have searched and I have hunted to prove that alcohol is harmful to the human anatomy. But I must . . . admit that I can come up with no clear-cut evidence that using alcohol in moderation does the human body the slightest bit of harm." [1]

"Moderate drinking" is hard to define. Even among those Dr. Pearl classed as moderate drinkers, the amount of consumption, of course, varied. But Dr. Pearl did say that a bottle of beer a day was within the bounds of moderation, so if you enjoy a little daily nip, it may be harmless.

However, despite the apparent harmlessness of moderate drinking, I must warn you that there are insidious dangers even in moderation. If you don't drink, it would be prudent not to start. A considerable portion of those who take up drinking eventually find that it becomes a more serious problem than they had anticipated. For them, drinking becomes a health-destroyer and a life-shortener.

According to varying estimates, the number of alcoholics in the United States is somewhere between six and a half million and sixteen million. This fact brings forth the startling statistic that perhaps one American in twenty is an alcoholic. This is a staggering figure (no pun intended), especially when allowance is made for all the nondrinkers. It would seem that anyone who imbibes runs a considerable risk of becoming an alcoholic. Moreover, many people become problem drinkers who, though not outright alcoholics, nevertheless have a habit that will damage their health and shorten their life.

For some people, even moderate drinking may be ex-

1 *The Provoker*, November-December 1969.

cessive. After I came across Dr. Pearl's findings, I resumed the enjoyment of an evening bottle of beer or a glass of wine. But I stopped a few months later when I developed a severe attack of gout. I decided that I was one of the people who should avoid alcohol even in moderation. As Dr. Pearl warns: "Individual tolerance for alcohol is a highly variable phenomenon . . . a conclusion which is on the average true for a large statistical aggregate may not be so for a particular individual in that aggregate." [2]

I have told you that the two leading fatal diseases are heart disease and cancer. You may have wondered which disease holds the dishonorable distinction of ranking third. It is alcoholism, which only now is being recognized as a disease. Take care not to catch it.

Medicines, with their harmful chemicals, should seldom, if ever, be needed by the conscientious follower of healthful living practices. Pursuing the program advocated in these pages can make pills and medicines unnecessary, or nearly so.

Drinking water that has been treated with chemicals can be avoided by either of two alternatives. One popular way is to draw water from a spring which has been tested for purity. If you can find such a source nearby, an occasional trip to it will keep you supplied with water for both drinking and cooking. Store this water in your refrigerator.

An easier way to insure pure drinking water is the installation of one of the filters sold by health-food dealers. Attached to your faucet, such a filter will remove chemicals from the water passing through it.

By now it should be clear to you that you can't entirely

[2] Raymond Pearl, *Alcohol and Longevity* (New York: A.A. Knopf, 1926).

escape the poisons being thrown at you from all sides, no matter how hard you try. However, the chemicals you can't avoid can be neutralized to some extent.

Detoxifying the poisons that have entered your body is the job of your liver. A healthy liver will eliminate a certain amount of the poisons you take in before they can do any harm. The health of your liver and that of your other organs can be improved if you follow the practices outlined in this book.

Probably the best way to promote the health of your liver is to feed it those elements it needs. These are Vitamin E and the entire family of B Vitamins. Rich in B vitamins, as well as in another yet-unidentified substance which helps to protect the body against poisons, is liver, so to keep your liver healthy, *eat* liver.

Another food element helps to combat chemicals by somehow acting to neutralize or detoxify them. This substance is Vitamin C. Therefore, to help your body overcome the poisons you can't avoid, get plenty of liver, Vitamin E, and Vitamin C.

SUMMARY

To reduce intake of poisonous spray residue in and on produce, eat fruits and vegetables with thick, inedible outer coverings, eat vegetables that grow underground, avoid or curtail intake of the fruits and vegetables that are sprayed most heavily, eat seed foods, and soak leafy vegetables and fruits with edible skins in a poison-removing solution and rinse them in cold running water.

To avoid poisonous spray residues completely, eat organically grown fruits and vegetables, eat ocean fish in place of meat, and avoid shellfish and fish from inland waterways.

To avoid or reduce the intake of poisonous food additives, buy foods without additives from health-food dealers, and when buying from other sources, check labels to avoid foods that have been heavily treated with chemicals.

To reduce your intake of polluted air, move to a relatively unpolluted area, if possible; if not, spend time in the country whenever you can.

To avoid or reduce the intake of miscellaneous other poisons, either don't smoke or switch to a pipe or cigars, drink alcoholic beverages only in moderation or avoid them entirely, avoid medicine whenever possible, and drink either pure spring water or install a filter on your drinking faucet.

To help your body neutralize the poisons you can't avoid, eat liver and Vitamins E and C.

twenty-two

The Technocrats

The bad thing about the poison deluge is that the worst is yet to come.

Looking back at the recent past, it is obvious from the vast increase in technological developments that the coming decades will see bigger and worse threats to man's health and existence. At the rate we are now progressing, the present age may soon be looked upon as the "good old days."

To the dangers already present, new ones are certain to be added, for behind the ever-growing list of hazards to human health and life is the fact that man's knowledge is increasing at a rapidly accelerating rate. We are experiencing a technological revolution unlike anything the world has seen.

Ninety percent of all the scientists the world has ever known, are living today. Of all the money spent on research and development since our country was founded, about half has been invested in the past ten years. A drug company ad boasts that "90% of today's prescriptions could not have been filled as recently as ten years ago."

Food additives are being discovered faster than they can be adequately tested.

The frighteningly accelerating rate of increase in scientific and technical knowledge is emphatically brought home by figures from the magazine *The Plain Truth*, which says: "The amount of knowledge which it took man from the birth of Jesus Christ to 1750 to acquire was doubled between 1750 and 1900—in just 150 years. Between 1900 and 1950 man's knowledge doubled again—this time in only 50 years. And in the one short decade between 1950 and 1960 it doubled yet again!" [1]

Today, the knowledge boom is being accelerating at an even faster rate. To quote again from *The Plain Truth*: "Knowledge is now estimated to be doubling every two and one-half years. By 1975, man's fund of accumulated knowledge will double *every three months*—if present trends continue!"

As we have already learned, when our knowledge increases, so do our physical troubles. In the near future, new and bigger troubles will descend upon us at a faster and faster rate.

Some future technological developments will be for the better, but many others will be for the worse. Some new inventions and processes are sure to create disastrous side effects that will far outweigh their benefits. This will happen because a tremendous gap often exists between finding new knowledge and putting it to proper use. The brain of man has more creative power than good judgment. Man cannot resist snatching small short-term gain at the risk of great long-term loss.

Just around the corner, all kinds of ominous innovations are lurking. On the drawing boards or already in experimental stages are many potential menaces, such as drugs to boost human intelligence, chemicals to convert weeds

[1] *The Plain Truth*, February, 1969.

into edible foods, the growth of vegetables without soil, preservation of foods by irradiation, governing the sex of unborn children, and electric sleep, which will enable people to get by on two hours sleep a night. Far-sighted observers warn of the delayed and dire side effects of such developments.

Nuclear power is another technological development against which we are being warned. Larry Bogart, director of the Anti-Pollution League in Allendale, New Jersey, writes in a letter to *Life* magazine: "The greatest pollution yet is being prepared for America. It's called 'clean' energy from nuclear power plants. With radioactive pollution you can have a clean environment—clean of living things." [2]

I first became aware of environmental chemicals and their unhealthful consequences in the late 1940's. In those days, the few who warned against the growing menace were dismissed as extremists or crackpots. Today, more than twenty years later, I have the satisfaction of witnessing these once-derided dangers being officially recognized and commonly acknowledged. I hope to live long enough to see even greater progress in the war upon technology's bogus benefits. I hope to witness an age in which all new technology is viewed with suspicion. I hope to see the day when short-range benefits that appear desirable are carefully weighed against potential long-term disadvantages.

For the protection of health and life, measures must be set up to police the technocrats. The first tentative steps in this direction are now being taken. Both the House and the Senate are currently considering the establishment of bodies to assess new developments in technology.

The question that arises is why the government doesn't do more to protect us against the ever-multiplying menaces to health and life. Why aren't poisoners denied their

[2] *Life*, February 28, 1969.

contaminants? Why are refiners permitted to steal vital nutrients from our foods? Why doesn't our government do more to restrain technological overkill?

The reason the government doesn't do more to protect you and me is that too many lawmakers are too often being dominated by the interests of big business.

More than two thousand organizations, most of which are connected with big business, are spending over a billion dollars a year in what are often successful attempts to influence legislation. To get the laws they favor passed, these special-interest groups send lobbyists to the capitol to wheedle, pressure, and intimidate our lawmakers. When legislation is pending which concerns the food industry, tobacco growers, chemical manufacturers, or air polluters, you can bet that their lobbyists are hard at work, trying to sway the lawmakers. Legislators usually hear far more from the small minorities who are looking out for their own selfish interests than they do from the vast majority of our population.

Most legislators, however, even if only for their own good, want to represent the views of the majority who elected them to office, for their voting power can make or break these legislators.

How can you and I reach and influence our lawmakers? With a powerful little eight-cent stamp and a little time. If a citizen feels strongly enough on a subject to sit down and write a letter about it, the lawmaker has to notice it. Legislators usually pay little heed to petitions or form letters. Signatures are easy to get, and many of them have little meaning. The personal letter is the one which carries the most weight.

Lobbyists present *reasons* for their viewpoint on controversial matters. They may try to show that despite the possible harm to public health that would result from passing or not passing a particular law, the opposite might hurt business and consequently create unemployment which would, in turn, disrupt the economy.

The eight-cent lobbyist must show the other side of the argument and tell the lawmaker not only what he is for or against, but also *why*.

The address of the President is: The White House, Washington, D. C. 20501; of your two senators: The Senate Office Building, Washington, D. C. 20510; and of your representative: The House Office Building, Washington, D. C. 20515.

On the state level, you can write to the governor of your state and your two congressmen in care of your state capitol building.

If you don't know the names of your elected officials, you can get them from the headquarters of your local political organization, your election board, or the offices of the League of Women Voters.

If you sometimes feel you want to reach a representative faster than you could by letter, you can do so simply by picking up your phone. Western Union has a special political-message service, called the "Personal Opinion Message." The company will send your fifteen-word telegram to the President, or to a congressman, governor, or state legislator at a special low rate. This charge is then added to your phone bill. If you don't know a representative's name, Western Union will look it up for you.

After election day, continue using the power of your vote by letting lawmakers know where you stand on matters affecting your health. In the long run, the best way to fight public pollution is to influence our legislators so that they stop poisons at their sources.

SUMMARY

To help stop the many forms of public poisoning at their sources, send your arguments against them to our lawmakers.

twenty-three

The Forgotten Art

Perhaps it was surprising to you to discover that some health-conscious individuals deliberately miss a meal now and then and that they can do so not only without ill effects, but also to the benefit of their health. If you did find this surprising, what comes next may prove flabbergasting.

Some of the wise few believe in doing completely without food for periods that range from a day or two to many weeks, as a health measure. During the entire fast they take nothing but water. The reason they fast is to give their bodies an opportunity to be cleansed of impurities. Freed of the task of digesting, assimilating, and metabolizing food, the body has a chance to clean house.

When you stop feeding your body, it becomes dependent upon the nutrition you have stored. When using up stored nutrients, your system also carries stored toxins to the organs of elimination. Long-retained waste is eliminated. As the fast continues, the body is completely cleansed. The fast is a period of purification and rejuvenation.

One reason Bernarr Macfadden probably far outlived
the others in his family was the many fasts with which he
cleansed and rejuvenated his body.

Eighty-nine-year-young Paul Bragg fasts several times
a year, for periods of a week to ten days. In addition, he
fasts one day each week.

Richard Condon, the author, fasted for two weeks at a
health farm, lost twenty-eight pounds, and reduced his
blood pressure considerably. He said: "I never felt better
in my life," and he wrote an enthusiastic book on the subject, *The Pleasures of Fasting* (Random House).

Many of the oldsters in the Gallup survey fasted when
they were sick. Dr. Gallup quotes one of them as saying,
"When I don't feel up to snuff, I just starve myself for a
few days and that fixes me up."

Fasting's advocates agree that this treatment is particularly necessary when the need for purification is indicated by illness. As proof, they offer the evidence that
during illness the human body usually loses its desire for
food and that animals stop eating when they get sick.
The desire for liquids continues, but appetite for food is
strongly diminished or completely lacking. This loss of
appetite is apparently the body's way of asking for a rest,
to pave the way for necessary repair work.

When an animal gets sick, it finds a quiet, secluded spot
where it can rest undisturbed while its body carries on
the work of restoring health. Man believes, however, that
he must continue eating during illness. Man, who does not
trust nature and feels he knows better than nature, force-
feeds himself to keep up his strength, and thereby weakens
himself even more.

One proponent of fasting comments: "It is a popular
idea that man is immediately and utterly dependent upon
food supplies every few hours, and that he will grow weak
and die if he misses a few meals. Well or sick, we are expected to eat three or more times each day. We are to be

deaf, blind, and silent to every signal of distress, and eat in spite of such signals. If there is no desire for food, eat anyway; if there is actual repugnance for food, disregard it; if there is nausea, eat; if the digestive function is badly impaired or has been suspended so that digestion is impossible, eat anyway. Such is the popular misconception." [1]

During the past forty-five years, Dr. Shelton has convinced more than thirty thousand of his patients to make fasts of varying length. Although many of the fasts lasted only a few days, some continued for much longer periods, and many lasted for more than sixty days. Two of Dr. Shelton's patients fasted for seventy days, and the longest fast of all lasted an amazing ninety days.

Dr. Shelton, and other advocates of fasting, point to many cases of alleviation or cure of disease by means of temporary fasts. Name almost any ailment, and the record will show examples of its relief or remedy as a result of the nonmedical measure of fasting.

George S. Weger, M.D., head of the Weger Health School in Redlands, California, who is an experienced exponent of fasting, writes: "Nothing is more gratifying, no work more inspiring, than actually to witness complete recovery during comparatively short periods of fasting in diseases such as chronic eczema, urticaria of years' standing, varicose ulcers, gastric and duodenal ulcers, asthma, arthritis, colitis, amoebic dysentery, endocarditis, sinusitis, bronchitis, neuritis, Bright's disease, acute and chronic appendicitis, tic douloureux, fistula, psoriasis, all kinds of digestive disorders, urinary and biliary caluli, pellagra, glaucoma, lump on the breast, epithelioma, migraine, acidosis, pupura hemorrhagica, epilepsy, paralysis agitans, Reyaud's disease . . ." [2]

---

[1] Herbert M. Shelton, *Fasting Can Save Your Life* (Chicago: Natural Hygiene Press, Inc.).

[2] *Ibid.*

Most impressive of the cures wrought by fasting are cases that doctors had previously given up as incurable. In addition, there is a great deal of convincing evidence of fasting's power to *prevent* disease.

In spite of fasting's history of cure and rejuvenation and despite its obvious effectiveness in disease prevention, the art of fasting is today all but forgotten. This old-fashioned health technique is ignored by the new school of nutritionists, who accent eating rather than not eating. Supplying the body with an abundance of nutrients is considered by many to be the sole dietary secret of keeping fit.

No one can deny that a nutritious diet is one of the main ways to promote good health, but evidence shows that health may also be protected, improved, and even restored by periods of abstention from all food.

Did early man fast? He must have, although it was probably unintentional. In nature, food is not always plentiful. Wild animals must get by at times on reduced food intake, or even do without it, as is sometimes shown by their springtime gauntness. Primitive man must also have experienced lean intervals. Times of plenty were almost certainly interspersed with periods of scarcity or even famine. Sometimes early man feasted, but sometimes he fasted. He set a pattern for us to follow.

SUMMARY

A few times a year, help your body to detoxify by fasting, particularly if a need to do so is indicated by minor illness.

twenty-four

Health the Fast Way

Ready to try a fast? Even a short one can clear debris from your cells, rejuvenate your body, and make you feel like a new person. Provided you are in good health, it can do you no harm to undergo a short fast without medical supervision; on the contrary, it can do you a world of good. If your doctor certifies that you are free from organic defect, you can safely fast for as long as three days.

If you decide to fast, you will want to know certain things. Probably the question most often asked of those who have fasted is "How could you stand the hunger pangs?"

During a fast there is usually surprisingly little sensation of hunger. At the beginning of the fast—for the first day or so—there is the feeling of hunger that is normally felt at mealtime, but as the fast progresses, this feeling subsides. While fasting, I have frequently sat at the dinner table with my family without having the slightest desire for food.

During a fast, the intake of drinking water must continue, for water is needed to help carry off accumulated toxins, and it is, of course, also necessary to life itself.

Authorities on fasting recommend that physical activity be kept to a minimum. Some advise going to bed and staying there, except for trips to the bathroom; others permit a little light activity. But it is generally agreed that exercise interferes with purification, while rest accelerates this process.

Bathing or showering is permitted and may aid the eliminative process, in fact. But the bath or shower should be of short duration.

Short sun baths are also permitted during a fast, but long exposure to the sun should be avoided.

The faster should keep comfortably warm. Excessive cold can prove enervating and thus hinder the purification process.

During even a short fast, bowel movements are reduced or cease entirely.

A few mildly disagreeable symptoms may be noticed during a fast. The tongue may become coated and an unpleasant taste in the mouth may develop. Headache or other aches may be experienced. These symptoms should create no alarm. They are good signs—indications that the purification process is proceeding as it should.

At the conclusion of a fast, eating should be resumed gradually. Don't overburden your system suddenly with a heavy meal. I suggest you start with a piece or two of fruit or some fruit juice, following this a few hours later with something a bit more substantial. Your first few meals should be small ones. Don't throw your body into high gear too abruptly.

Another warning I must issue to anyone who fasts concerns a pair of hazards which didn't exist some years ago, but which exist in the poisoned world of today. These new hazards are caused by our civilization's backward progress. They are the result of pesticides and strontium. Pesticides have been used in such enormous quantities that today they are even found in polar regions. Strontium in vast quantities has been discharged into the world atmosphere by the testing of atom bombs. These two kinds of poison have found their way into every human body in America, including yours.

Pesticides have an affinity for the body's fatty tissues. When you fast, your body uses stored fat as fuel. As the fat enters the blood, it brings stored pesticides with it, which poison your bloodstream.

Strontium gravitates toward the bones. The effect of fasting on strontium is to drive it deeper into the bones.

Can anything be done to eliminate or minimize these modern hazards?

An effective agent for helping the body eliminate poisons is Vitamin C. Taking a Vitamin C tablet or a glass of orange juice every now and then during a fast will help eliminate pesticides from the bloodstream.

Of course, when a fast is interrupted by the intake of citrus fruit juice or a Vitamin C supplement, it is no longer a true fast. But such a small intake is not enough to interfere seriously with the body's eliminative processes. (Some modern fasters take multiple vitamin supplements while fasting and get good results.)

My most-recent fasts were accomplished by using Vitamin C as a detoxifier. Three or four times a day at widely spaced intervals, I drank a glass of freshly squeezed orange juice.

I don't know what effect Vitamin C may have on the strontium in your system. I wish I could tell you that Vitamin C or some other substance would help eliminate this dastardly poison, but I haven't been able to find any evidence to that effect.

One or two fasts may bring you such noticeable health improvement and rejuvenation that you will become a fasting zealot, as have others before you. But don't let your enthusiasm carry you away. Although fasting can be curative, health-building, and even life-saving, too-often-repeated fasting can prove harmful. For most people, a few times a year is sufficient.

If you enjoy eating as much as I do, you won't like to fast. I feel little hunger during a fast, but I keenly miss the pleasure of eating. Even though I know from experience that a fast will make me feel better and will noticeably improve my health, I embark on a fast with reluctance.

However, I find it very easy to fast for part of a day each week. I just skip breakfast and lunch. I don't mind fasting all day if I can look forward to a meal in the evening. This weekly, two-meal fast, brief though it is, often brings benefits that I can notice immediately.

None of my advice on meal-skipping or fasting is applicable to pregnant or nursing mothers or to growing children. Occasional meal-skipping or even short fasts might be advisable in some circumstances, but this should be left to a doctor's judgment.

In the presence of certain ailments, such as gout, experts warn that fasting may do more harm than good. However, I once ignored these warnings, with good results, I think.

During one gout attack, I underwent my longest fast, one that lasted for a week. This was easy, because the pain from my gout eliminated any desire for food. Thereafter, I enjoyed freedom from gout for four blessed years—my longest gout-free period, and during the following four years, I suffered only minor attacks.

Although it is true that an extended fast sometimes brings on gout, this may be the result of toxic substances being removed from the body as a result of fasting. Gout originates because a metabolic defect hinders normal expulsion of the uric acid formed in the human body. By initiating the process of toxin elimination, perhaps fasting also causes uric acid to leave the body. The movement of excess sharp uric-acid crystals toward the point of elimination causes the intense pain of gout.

I have just suffered my first severe siege of gout since the week-long fast, so perhaps it is once again time for seven days of fasting. But all this is theory, for a single case proves nothing, so I'm not recommending a fast during a gout attack.

Furthermore, I must warn you against the misuse of fasting as self-treatment of any disease. Despite fasting's record of cure, its use in disease treatment should be attempted, if at all, only on the advice of a doctor, and under his supervision. If you suffer from an ailment which you think might be relieved or cured by fasting, consult a doctor. Try to find one who understands and is sympathetic to the art of fasting and is experienced in its techniques.

SUMMARY

To fast, you should continue your intake of drinking water, take Vitamin C several times each day, keep physical activity to a minimum, bathe or shower only briefly, and keep warm. Resume eating gradually.

Don't fast on your own, unless you are in good health, and then not for more than three days, and don't fast more than a few times a year. Don't use fasting for attempted self-treatment of disease except with the approval of your doctor.

twenty-five

The Well Adjusted

While searching for the physical causes of poor health and abbreviated life span, I kept running into a strange and frustrating fact. Only one-third of those sick enough to seek a doctor's services suffer from illness that has a purely physical cause. The ailments of the remaining two-thirds are wholly or at least partly of *mental* origin. Mental and emotional tribulations are behind two out of every three cases of illness. The percentage is put even higher by some doctors, who estimate that emotional causes contribute to as much as 90% or more of all illness.

Because the emotions are heavily involved in so many cases of unnecessary sickness and untimely death, I place this health and longevity factor even before proper nutrition.

That emotions are capable of producing bodily reactions is easily demonstrated. The effect of an emotion is sometimes immediate and obvious. Shame or embarrassment may cause blushing. Fear can cause the skin to perspire, and in extreme cases, the entire body to tremble. Emotional conflict can produce skin eruptions, as in hives, the classic example.

At the same time that these *outwardly* visible reactions to emotional agitation are taking place, corresponding reactions take place *within* the body. Tests show that, during emotional stress, the heart rate and blood pressure rise, chemical composition of the blood alters, and other internal changes take place.

Even more-complex chemical and physiological alterations take place within the body when emotional stress is severe and of long duration. These stress reactions can bring on illness, or at least make a person more susceptible to it.

Onset of the common cold, as has been demonstrated time and time again, can be triggered by emotional upheaval. Dr. Merl M. Jackel, a psychoanalyst and senior lecturer in the division of psychoanalytic education at the State University of New York, is one expert who has observed that colds can begin in the mind. Dr. Jackel studied cold incidence in ten of his patients over a period of three years. Out of twenty-six colds, all but one followed a state of depression.

That colds are induced by emotions rather than germs is endorsed by English psychiatrist Dr. E. W. Braithwaite, consulting psychiatrist to the Ministry of Health, who says: ". . . the solution of the problem of the common cold lies in the sphere of psychological medicine. The specific factor is psychological; the microbic one secondary." [1]

Not only colds, but also stomach ulcers, arthritis, diabetes, asthma, colitis, high blood pressure, and migraine headache are among the ailments commonly acknowledged as being often induced, at least in part, by psychosomatic causes.

Another ailment that can apparently be triggered by mental turmoil is gout, my own nemesis. Many gout vic-

[1] *British Medical Journal*, October 2, 1944.

tims, myself among them, have noticed that attacks seem to follow emotional stress.

Two other maladies often thought to be connected with emotional stress are the two leading causes of death: heart disease and cancer.

That heart health can be affected by emotional tension has been demonstrated by research numerous times. In a study of one hundred young heart-disease patients, conducted by Dr. Henry I. Russek, cardiovascular consultant to the United States Public Health Service Hospital on Staten Island, it was found that most of the sufferers had been subjected to unusual occupational stress just before their heart attacks. Ninety-one percent had been working long hours, sometimes at two jobs, or had suffered exceptionally from job-related feelings of fear, inadequacy, insecurity, or discontent.

Cancer is also often linked with emotional stress by professional observers. One expert who has noticed a relationship between emotional upheaval and cancer is Sir Heneage Ogilvie, famed British surgeon, who puts it thus in his book *No Miracles Among Friends*: "The instances when the first recognizable onset of cancer has followed almost immediately on some disaster, a bereavement, the break-up of a relationship, a financial crisis, or an accident, are so numerous that they suggest that some controlling force that has hitherto kept this outbreak of cell communism in check has been removed." [2]

J. I. Rodale found enough material on the close relationship between emotional state of mind and cancer to fill an entire book, which he titled *Happy People Rarely Get Cancer*.

Negative emotions like worry, fear, anxiety, apprehen-

[2] Sir Heneage Ogilvie, *No Miracles Among Friends* (London: Maxfield Parrish, 1959).

sion, and discouragement create mental turmoil and retard health and longevity. Positive emotions like cheerfulness, hope, serenity, and satisfaction create mental tranquility and promote health and longevity.

Once they understand that negative emotions can cause sickness, some practical individuals are able to thrust these demons from their minds. One man I know virtually eliminated worry from his life in this way. He had for some time been under a pile of stressful situations. A professional man, he had made the down payment on a building to house both his office and his living quarters, but his volume of business turned out to be less than he had expected. In addition, he had trouble collecting delinquent accounts. Then he discovered that the old structure he had bought required more in the way of repairs and modernization than he had anticipated. In an attempt to increase his income, he opened a second office in another city, thus adding still more tension. My friend had a bull by the tail and couldn't let go.

But a visit from his brother, who happened to be a doctor, straightened him out. Although the doctor did nothing to alleviate his brother's troubles, he was able to show him the possible consequences of worrying about them. "He opened my eyes to what worry can do to your health," said my friend. "It can actually make you sick and cause serious diseases, even cancer. I've quit worrying. It's not worth it."

Another fellow I talked with has developed the same philosophy. "My brother died of ulcers," he told me. "The doctors said that worry caused them. Now I don't worry about anything."

Like the two men I have just told you about, some people who have acquired the bad habit of harboring negative emotions can suddenly break away from them. But for most of us, the technique of substituting good for bad emotions takes time to learn. Of all the many health and longevity factors, mental tranquility can be the hardest to put into permanent practice. But you can do it, because others are doing so.

Some people meet every problem in life with good emotions. In the face of life's inevitable ups and downs, these well-adjusted people usually manage to carry on with optimism, good cheer, and mental tranquility. Even when faced with intolerable situations, these compliant individuals respond for the most part by ignoring, adjusting to, or accepting the circumstances.

Other people, frequently with less cause, meet life's inescapable vicissitudes with fear, worry, apprehension, and discouragement.

How can you become one of the better-adjusted individuals who promotes his health with mental tranquility? By learning to govern your thinking. You can control your thoughts more than anything else in this world. Whenever you find yourself entertaining negative thoughts, try to replace them with emotions like serenity, hope, and cheerfulness. Just as you replaced deficient, health-destroying foods with wholesome, healthful foods, you must replace negative, health-destroying emotions with wholesome, healthful emotions.

As you strive to replace hurtful emotions with healthful ones, you must allow for possible temporary setbacks. Just when you have been making progress, a situation may come along that knocks your emotions into a tailspin. You must then return, albeit slowly, to replacing your bad emotions with good ones.

With practice, you may become one of those lucky humans who are largely free from the damaging effects of mental turmoil, a well-adjusted individual who refrains from polluting his body with the poisons created by emotional ferment.

Summary

Emotional stress can contribute to illness. Practice replacing harmful emotions like worry, fear, anxiety, apprehension, and discouragement with healthful emotions like cheerfulness, hope, serenity, and satisfaction.

twenty-six

Help Yourself

Negative emotions provoke disease; positive emotions promote health. Help yourself attain health-conserving, life-lengthening emotional quietude with the seven tips that follow.

1. WHEN YOU FEEL GOOD, BE HAPPY

Somewhere I read about a man who feels happy most of the time. It's not that this man has any more to be happy about than the average person. He is happy because of the attitude he has adopted. His philosophy is: "On any day that I am reasonably free of physical or mental pain, I should be happy. I can't always have everything going exactly the way I want it. I can't always be having a wildly exciting time. But on the days when I am free or nearly free from physical or mental pain, I have much to be thankful for."

This man is usually happy because he knows what is really important, and he is grateful when he has it. His philosophy would be an excellent one for anyone to adopt, especially the person who seeks and appreciates good health.

2. LOOK ON THE BRIGHT SIDE

A young man who always seems to be smiling and cheerful told me the secret of his contentment. He said: "I can look at the people going by and see someone better off than me, but I can also see someone who is worse off than me. I have formed the habit of comparing my lot with that of the fellow worse off than I am. Thus, even when things don't go entirely to my liking, I still feel happy."

When you need an antidote for your troubles and discouragements, just consider for a moment someone who is worse off than you are. And when things go wrong, remember that they could be worse. In every situation, there is something for which to be thankful. If you make a bad business deal, remember that many have made worse. If you wreck your car, think of someone who wrecked his and was killed in the process.

The wise man forms the habit of comparing his lot with those who have less and of looking on the bright side of every situation.

3. PROBLEMS USUALLY WORK OUT

The professional man I told you about who had banished worry from his mind found that his troubles gradually disappeared. As he went along from day to day doing the best he could and not worrying, things gradually began to look up.

When problems are faced with equanimity, they usually get solved just as well as they would if they were handled with desperation—sometimes even better. Seemingly insurmountable problems often have a way of working out or eventually turning out to be minor or nonexistent.

Mark Twain put all this into a few wise and witty words. If my memory is correct, they went like this: "I am an old man who has seen many troubles, most of which never happened."

4. EVERYONE IS IN THE SAME BOAT

No one's life is a bed of roses, even though it sometimes seems that a chosen few have all the luck. But even the luckiest, wealthiest, best-looking, most-famous people suffer frustrations, disappointments, failures, and worries.

Rabbi Joshua Liebman, in his book *Peace of Mind*, put it this way: "The neurotic thinks that everything happens to him. He fails to see that it also happens to his sisters, brothers, friends, and, yes, even to the President." [1]

When the going gets rough, remember that you have plenty of company. No one's life is all smooth sailing. Everyone has his share of troubles, cares, and burdens, but life is kindest to those with mental serenity, natural or acquired.

5. LOWER YOUR DAILY GOALS

Many of us are in a hurry today. We have too much to do and not enough time to do it. The urgency to get things done is responsible for much present-day tension.

I sometimes fall into the hurry-worry trap myself. When I begin work in the morning, it is often with the idea of completing certain tasks by the day's end. If some phases of the work don't go well or if I am bothered by interruptions, I may find myself falling behind schedule. It is then easy to start getting tense.

But I have learned that if I set a lower goal for myself each day, I can then take the slow-downs and interruptions in stride. With an easier goal, pressure is removed. I prob-

[1] Joshua Liebman, *Peace of Mind* (New York: Simon and Schuster, Inc., 1946).

ably get as much done, perhaps more, with less wear and tear on my nervous system.

Don't try to do too much too fast. This tip is from *To-day's Health*: "Take it easy, do your best, and what you do will be good enough."

6. LOWER YOUR OVERALL GOALS

If you find life dominated by mental stress, it is time to pause and take stock, to step back and examine your life to see what is causing your mental turmoil. Tracking down the tension-causers may enable you to overhaul your life and simplify it. Perhaps the cause of your emotional stress can be modified in some way or even expunged entirely from your life.

Careful examination of your way of life may reveal that one facet of your life is causing much of your mental conflict. It might be a job you dislike, which can be changed —even though it may mean a sacrifice in pay. It might be heavy living expenses, which can perhaps be trimmed by settling for less in the way of worldly goods. Whatever it is that is causing your mental gymnastics, it can perhaps be eliminated or changed.

In modern-day America, the basic reason for much mental and emotional conflict is the pursuit of money and status.

The status seeker often lives with perpetual mental stress. Such an individual sets high goals for himself. He seeks advancement in his job or business. He wants a pretentious home in the "right" suburb. He craves an expensive car. His children must attend one of the "best" colleges. He must belong to the "proper" clubs.

Reaching his goal often fails to satisfy the seeker of wealth and status. By the time he attains the success at which he aims, he has probably already readjusted his sights toward still higher achievement.

The insatiable striver for wealth and status allows his sense of values to get distorted. He has his priorities mixed up. Achieving a goal in life is not a matter of life or death, but its pursuit may well be. The man who is successful at the cost of health and life is a successful failure.

7. GUILT FEELINGS

Worry, apprehension, fear, and other such feelings are not the only kinds of emotions that are destructive to health. Another such emotion is the feeling of *guilt*.

Most of us were brought up to follow certain standards of behavior. In the home, school, and church, we were taught self-discipline. A strong sense of right and wrong is deeply implanted early in life. We are expected to live up to certain ideals. However, these high goals are not always attainable. When, through all-too-human frailties, we violate the ideals inculcated in us, we create within ourselves feelings of guilt.

Unfortunately, the matter doesn't end there. At the same time we were learning about right and wrong, we also learned that we must pay for wrongdoing. Therefore, when we feel that we have erred or fallen short of certain standards, we also feel a subconscious need to punish ourselves.

Psychologists know that self-punishment often takes various strange forms. One is the making of mistakes, sometimes foolish ones. Another is the losing of valuables.

But sometimes the punishment takes a more serious form, and it becomes a sickness. Through sickness, the person who feels guilty is "paying" for his "sins." The pain of illness atones for the feeling of guilt.

Ainslie Meares, M.D., in his book *Relief Without Drugs*, tells about the person who thus punishes himself. "In a sense he is glad of the pain. By suffering the pain he will ease his conscience of the thing that he has done, and his mind will be at rest again.

"On the one hand, a patient in this situation wants to get rid of the pain because it hurts him, but on the other hand, he wants to keep it, as it expiates his feelings of guilt." [2]

Of course, the sufferer is unaware of the connection between his guilt feelings and his illness. Indeed, he may not even be aware of his guilt feelings, but in his subconscious mind he still feels the need for punishment.

Some of the things that people feel guilty about were unearthed in a poll of American adults by public-opinion analyst Louis Harris. A few of the admitted causes of guilt feelings, as reported in the *Washington Post*, were: Ate more than should at a meal, am out of shape physically, do too little reading, don't go to church regularly, waste too much time, not considerate enough of parents, spend too much time watching TV, spend more money than I can afford, not considerate enough of children, drink too much for my own good.

Very few of those polled mentioned what is perhaps the leading cause of guilt feelings, the sex instinct.

Our earlier forebears were able to express this natural urge without qualms. But in our present-day society, sex is repressed, restricted, restrained, reproached, reviled, and if in any way expressed, often regretted. Yet the sexual instinct is a normal one, developed through the incalculable centuries of our evolution. Consider for a moment, if you will, your own evolutionary background.

If your genealogy could be traced to its origin, it would go back uninterrupted, all the way to the beginning of life on earth three hundred and fifty million years ago.

[2] Ainslie Meares, *Relief Without Drugs* (New York: Ace Books, Inc., 1967).

Through eons of time, your lineage never once faltered. Never did a single one of your ancestors fail to reach maturity and reproduce. Those of your forebears who swung from the trees, those who crawled on the ground before them, those who swam in the seas even before *them*—all found a mate and reproduced themselves. If just one pair of your ancestors—fish, reptile, animal, or human—sometime, somewhere in those millions of generations had failed to carry out the reproductive process and broken the chain, you wouldn't exist.

Is it any wonder that the sex instinct is strong? In much the same way that the human race has become dependent on certain food elements in its diet, it has also become conditioned to sex in its life. Surviving for innumerable generations on certain food elements has reinforced the need for them. Similarly, countless repetitions of the sex act have strengthened the sex urge. Sex desire is as normal as the desire for food; its lack would be abnormal.

But because of unapproved sex conduct of one kind or another, and sometimes because of the mere thought of it, some people bear a heavy burden of guilt feelings. The well-publicized inquiries of Dr. Alfred Kinsey into American sex practices brought a sigh of relief from many. One no-longer-tortured woman said: "No one has any idea of how much better it made me feel to learn that there were many other people like me."

All this is not to condone sex practices frowned upon by society, but to propose that a more realistic and understanding attitude is needed on the part of society. A more realistic and understanding attitude of the individual toward himself is also needed.

Another major cause of guilt feelings is *hostility* toward others. Feelings of hostility or hate can give rise to guilt feelings, particularly when they are directed against loved ones.

These feelings are sometimes consciously thought and expressed in words. The child may cry out "I hate you" or "I wish you were dead." More often, these feelings of hostility are repressed. Because we consciously reject such feelings, we unconsciously turn them inward. They may later emerge in the form of illness.

Man's capacity for hostility is another carry-over from his earlier days. Our ancestors wouldn't have survived long without an aggressive nature. The aggression we have inherited often ends up as forbidden feelings of hostility, which in turn bring on feelings of guilt and end up as physical sickness.

How can we successfully combat our feelings of guilt? What can we do to prevent or to minimize their damaging effects? First, we can strive to live virtuously. Because doing what we consider wrong is the cause of guilt feelings, we must try to do what we feel is right. We can thus lighten or remove the load of guilt. Leading an upright life helps promote a healthy mental attitude. We have all experienced the feeling of self-approval that follows a good deed.

But at the same time we are trying to practice virtue, we must also learn to forgive our errors. Church doctrine tells us that God forgives all those who are sincerely repentant. Why then should we not forgive ourselves?

SUMMARY

To help replace harmful emotions with beneficial emotions, adopt the philosophy of feeling happy whenever you are reasonably free of physical or mental pain, form the habit of comparing your lot with that of those who have less and look on the bright side of every situation, realize that most problems eventually work out, and that they will do so just as well when faced with equanimity as when handled with desperation. Realize that even the luckiest people have troubles. Set low daily goals for yourself. Simplify your life by tracking down and eliminating or modifying the causes of mental turmoil, and combat guilt feelings by living virtuously, but forgiving yourself for slip-ups.

twenty-seven

Take the Sting Out

Don't expect to be 100% successful in banishing negative emotions from your life. No one can avoid mental stress completely, nor should he expect to.

A certain amount of concern for oneself has always been necessary for survival. Throughout the ages, the man who lasted the longest has been the one who looked ahead, storing food for the future and arming himself against enemies, or building up his bank balance. A little constructive worry can sometimes be beneficial. For example, without some fear of poor health, you wouldn't practice the prevention of illness.

Nevertheless, even those mental stresses which are inevitable are potentially harmful. Can anything be done about these inescapable emotional pressures? Yes. Mental tensions can be discharged to a great extent and their health-damaging consequences at least partially canceled.

Here are six ways of relieving emotional tensions you don't avoid. They can help to take the sting out of those harmful emotions you can't avoid.

1. EXPRESS YOUR ANGER

The tensions caused by exasperation, aggravation, and frustration can sometimes be released on the spot. When something or someone angers you, patience is not always an imperative. Instead of bottling up your feelings, give vent to them sometimes. You'll release your pent-up emotions and feel better immediately.

If you have been a "meekling" who never blows up, you may be pleasantly surprised to discover that if you pop off occasionally, you not only will be forgiven, but will also win respect.

Whenever possible, practice a little self-expression, instead of trying to practice self-control.

2. DON'T HOLD BACK TEARS

Another way of discharging strong emotions is by crying. To the child, this form of relief comes easily and naturally. But as early in life as possible, we begin to wean the child, particularly the male, away from this means of releasing tension. Crying in certain situations is considered excusable for girls and even for grown women, but the adolescent and adult male has been conditioned to stifle his instinct to cry.

Many experts agree that withheld tears can later emerge as sickness. The adult male's acquired proclivity to choke back the lump in his throat is perhaps one reason why women outlive men.

Our culture needs to amend its code of behavior so as to permit men to release emotional tension by crying openly. Until such a change occurs in behavior, men should give vent to feelings of strong emotion by crying in privacy or in the company of an understanding friend.

3. PHYSICAL ACTIVITY

Still another harmless way to work off emotional stress is through physical activity. Almost any activity will do

—taking a walk, chopping wood, driving golf balls, or scrubbing the kitchen floor. Any physical outlet can help you work off tension. We'll discuss this further a little later.

4. TALK IT OUT

Often the best therapy for emotional tribulation is to talk problems out. In talking about your trouble, you may get rid of it by talking it out of you. Even if you don't succeed in ridding yourself of whatever is bothering you, you may at least minimize its importance.

When fears are brought into the open, they often shrink to manageable size. Tumbled about in your mind, a problem can appear insurmountable, but once expressed in words and discussed, it can dwindle to proportions with which you can cope.

Instead of keeping your troubles to yourself, find a sympathetic listener, such as a clergyman or friend. In addition to the relief you'll gain from talking about your problems, you will have the chance to get another person's viewpoint on them. From a different perspective, he may see things you can't see, and be able to offer you helpful advice.

5. THE NEED FOR CARE AND ATTENTION

Psychologists agree that sickness can be one way of getting care or attention.

The need to be cared for is a basic human hunger. A lonely person who yearns for affection may sometimes become ill, as a means of getting the attention he craves.

Good friends can help you satisfy your natural desire to be important to others. Cultivate one or more friends who give you the sympathetic comradeship you need and do the same for them.

There is a secret to making friends: If you want to be cared about, care about others. The way to win a friend is to be one.

6. THE NEED TO GIVE

There is yet another reason for giving care and attention to others. Rabbi Joshua Liebman calls it "an inner necessity to give love and to bestow affection upon the outer world."

Many people have discovered that the more interested they become in other people's problems, in offering advice or lending a sympathetic ear, the less concerned they are with their own troubles. By cheering someone else, they also cheer themselves; by doing a good turn for someone else, they do themselves incalculable good; by letting someone lean on them, they themselves become stronger.

NATURAL TRANQUILIZERS

In addition to the aforementioned means, you can get extra help in achieving mental serenity from another source: your diet. Three health foods mentioned earlier exert a soothing, calming effect on their consumers: Dolomite, brewer's yeast, and desiccated liver are natural tranquilizers.

Regular use of dolomite will soon bring about a constant state of tranquility that borders on euphoria. Taking dolomite is something like wearing rose-colored glasses. Life looks better. Problems appear smaller and minor irritations can be taken in stride.

In brewer's yeast and desiccated liver, the tranquilizing element is Vitamin B.

One of the B Vitamins, thiamine, was employed by nutritionist Dr. Tom Spies, to obtain amazing improvement in the condition of patients who needed tranquilization. "He treated 115 cases of timid, depressed, 'nervous' patients with thiamine," reports *If You Must Smoke*, a book by J. I. Rodale, "and the longest elapsed time between the first thiamine dose and a visible personality change was— pay attention to this—30 minutes. Not 30 days, but 30 minutes effected a complete and highly desirable change in personalities of 115 nervous wrecks, converting them to pleasant and cooperative people! If that isn't a nerve tonic, then nothing deserves the name." [1]

MENTAL TRANQUILITY AND THE LONG-LIVED

The influence of mental tranquility on health and longevity is shown by observation of the healthy and long-lived.

In rating the general states of their happiness throughout their lives, 95% of Dr. Gallup's oldsters considered that they had been either fairly happy or very happy. When asked whether their home lives had been peaceful and quiet, 94% replied affirmatively.

Regardless of whether their happiness was due to fortunate circumstances or to their naturally cheerful dispositions, the fact remains that the constitutions of these long-lived folks were not subjected greatly to the wear and tear of emotional turmoil.

The Hunzans also live lives of emotional stability. In their land, juvenile delinquency and divorce are almost unknown. Hunzans have no jails, no police, and no army, since they do not need them. It is little wonder that doctors are also virtually unneeded in such a land.

SUMMARY

To help discharge emotional tensions you can't avoid, express anger whenever possible, instead of bottling it up, express emotion through tears when you feel the need, discharge tensions through physical activity, and talk out your troubles. Cultivate one or more friends who will give you sympathetic comradeship, and give care and attention to others. Also use dolomite, brewer's yeast, and desiccated liver, the natural tranquilizing foods.

[1] J. I. Rodale, *If You Must Smoke* (New York: Pyramid Publications, Inc., 1968).

twenty-eight

The Head in the Sand

What is the leading cause of death among Americans under forty-four years of age? Is it cancer, or some form of heart disease? A disease of the young, such as scarlet fever? It is not even a disease. The leading cause of death in the under-forty-four group is *accidents*.

Until after middle age, disease isn't the main killer. The calamity most likely to take the life of a child, teen-ager, young adult, or the middle-aged person is an accident.

When I first learned that accidents were the leading cause of death among children, it gave me quite a jolt. I had been concentrating my efforts on guarding my children's lives against disease, only to discover that accidents were the greater risk.

Even for those over the age of forty-four, the danger from accidents is not lessened. The risk remains just as great, but by that time other factors have begun to take the place of accidents as the leading killer. By this time people have reached the age when they are more vulnerable to certain diseases. Nevertheless, among all age groups combined, accidents are the fourth leading cause of death.

Accidents kill more than one hundred thousand Americans each year. You can grasp the staggering magnitude of this figure if you compare it with the population of your city.

Accidents, like disease, often maim when they do not kill. Each year accidents permanently disable four times as many persons as they kill.

What can be done about the accident rate? Aren't accidents largely unpreventable? Aren't they mostly due to carelessness which, for the most part, is substantially preventable only in theory, or simply the result of being in the wrong place at the wrong time, which is impossible to prevent?

Not true. Accidents are seldom caused solely by carelessness or chance, for the astonishing truth about accidents is that most of them don't happen by accident. Experts in accident research have found that most so-called accidents are not accidents at all. Incredible as it sounds, most accidents are purposely caused by the person to whom they happen or by the person in control of the situation.

"It is the consensus of psychiatric opinion that there is almost no such thing as a real accident," says Dr. Jean Rosenbaum, president of the New Mexico Psychoanalytical Association. "The majority of accidents are caused by somebody's unconscious desire to hurt, or in extreme cases, to destroy themselves. In other words a death wish." [1]

The real cause of most accidents is similar to the real cause of much illness. The accident victim, like the person who is ill, may bring about his own misfortune as a means

---

[1] *National Enquirer*, September 28, 1969.

of self-punishment, as a way to get care or attention, or as a method of expressing hostility.

Of course, the person who suffers from an accident that has been self-induced is seldom, if ever, aware that the accident actually represented a desire to hurt himself. He believes that the accident just happened. What he fails to realize is that he was subconsciously looking for an accident because he was psychologically ready for it to happen. If he had failed to have one, the next opportunity might have served.

Some people are chronic victims of accidents. These repeaters demonstrate that accidents aren't necessarily the result of pure chance. It has been proved by many surveys that some individuals are accident-prone. A study of factory workers showed that one-fourth of the workers had two-thirds of the accidents. Among a group of bus drivers, 10% of them had 25% of the accidents.

Accident research has brought out an odd fact about the accident-prone. Compared to the non-accident-prone, they enjoy better health. I offer the following explanation of this. The true causes of most accidents and of many illnesses are the same: psychosomatic. The accident repeater discharges his hostilities and guilt feelings through accidents, and he therefore has less "need" to be ill.

In view of the facts regarding the cause of most accidents, I propose the following four-step program for accident prevention: (1) The first step in avoiding accidents is the awareness that most accidents represent a desire to hurt oneself, (2) The second step would then be to convince oneself of the folly of such self-harming action, (3) Then try to avoid potential accident situations insofar as possible, and (4) Discharge self-destructive tendencies in a harmless fashion through expression and action.

Although most of us can readily picture ourselves being struck down by disease, we somehow feel that accidents only happen to someone else. The person who seeks health and longevity must replace such a head-in-the-sand attitude with the realization that the next accident may happen to him or to his loved ones.

Accidents happen everywhere, but more than half of them occur on our streets and highways. Unfortunately, it is in auto accidents that those who seek self-punishment are most apt to punish others at the same time. The careful driver's best defense is to drive "defensively."

Accidents involving children most often happen on bad days, when everything seems to be going wrong. Safety experts state that nine-out-of-ten accidents to children occur when they and their mothers are under temporary stress. These same circumstances are usually present when accidental self-poisoning of children occurs. (The most common accidental poisoner of children is aspirin.) One expert advises that a mother should temporarily relax her standards and cut a few corners during periods of emotional stress.

Accident prevention must begin with the realization that accidents are usually not accidental.

Summary

The important steps in accident prevention: awareness that most accidents represent a desire to hurt oneself, convincing oneself of the folly of such self-harming action, avoiding potential accident situations, and discharging self-destructive tendencies harmlessly through expression and action.

twenty-nine

The Drivers and the Conductors

Among the many health and longevity factors, there is one that is more influential than all the rest. Even more important than mental tranquility or good nutrition is this leading secret of good health and longevity. In the lives of healthy oldsters, one common trait stands out. The healthy old-timers have lived lives of vigorous physical activity. Of the Gallup oldsters, 70% of the men had worked at hard physical labor, 39% as manual laborers and 31% as farmers. Among the Social Security centenarians, 80% had been farmers for at least part of their lives, and a study of Russian centenarians reveals that 77% had been manual laborers, 61% farmers, and 16% factory workers.

Among the Hunzans, hard work is the way of life, for it is necessary for survival. The Hunzans are farmers, but their rocky, mountainous land is poorly suited to agriculture. Growing enough food to live requires the arduous labor of nearly everyone in Hunza. During the spring and summer, entire families work seven long days a week. Moreover, the Hunzans have no vehicles, so they must walk back and forth between their homes and the fields, which are usually located some distance away. Walking is also the only means of travel between the villages, which are ten to fifteen miles apart.

All these hard-working, healthy oldsters were following in the footsteps of their ancestors. For two million years, people had to expend considerable muscular energy in order to survive. As gatherers of wild foods and pursuers of wild game, our early forebears lived lives of vigorous physical activity. In this way, the human constitution, through countless generations of survival, became adapted to exercise.

Even after man gave up food-gathering and hunting, he didn't give up strenuous activity. Farming meant long hours of physical toil. Entire families formerly worked the land, much as the Hunzans do today.

Until the past few generations, people lived by laboring. Your parents or grandparents, in their earlier days at least, probably led a life far more strenuous than yours. In their day, convenience had not yet curtailed activity. Even those who earned their livelihood through sedentary work were far from inactive. The typical clerk or schoolmaster walked to and from his job. He also chopped wood, beat rugs, and spaded his garden. In summer, he pushed a lawnmower; in the winter, a snow shovel. His wife washed clothes by hand, pushed a broom, scrubbed floors on her knees, and went shopping on foot.

Today, all this has changed. The early 1900's saw a beginning of the decline in physical activity. Machinery began to replace muscle, and people began to take life easier. Gradually, they even walked less and less, and as a consequence, hearts and circulatory systems began to deteriorate from lack of exercise.

During the same years when food refining began to have ill effects on American heart health, further harm was being brought about by the national decline in activity.

At the same time that our foods have been virtually stripped of Vitamin E and other elements needed for heart health, at the same time that heart-damaging refined sugar has become a staple in our diets, the problem has been gravely compounded by lack of exercise. Small wonder that there is a heart disease "epidemic" in America today. Twelve million people are currently suffering from heart and artery disease. Each year, nearly one million persons die from these disorders. Heart disease has become the leading killer, and it now accounts for more than half of all deaths.

Until recently, the theory that physical activity protects the health of the heart was endorsed by only a few, but several years ago proof of this began to be uncovered. A 1953 report shattered the notion that activity was harmful to the heart, while rest was beneficial to it. This study compared thirty-one thousand drivers and conductors of London double-decker buses. The drivers sat still all day, of course, while the conductors walked back and forth in the aisles, climbed up and down the stairs, and stepped out at stops.

The drivers and conductors were equal in age and had the same eating habits. The only significant difference between the two groups was in their physical activity. The sedentary drivers were found to suffer more than twice as many heart attacks as the more active conductors. The sitters who were "saving" their hearts turned out to be more than twice as subject to heart attacks as their mobile counterparts whose hearts were being "worn out."

Since this pioneering survey, many others have compared the active and the inactive. Studies have compared farmers and townspeople, postal clerks and mail carriers, railroad clerks and section hands, athletes who continued exercise and those who didn't, heart patients who walked and those who indulged in little activity. Results have always been the same. The more activity, the less heart trouble; the less activity, the more heart trouble.

There can be no doubt that heart trouble is a disease of twentieth century American civilization. Although the incidence of heart disease has soared in America since the early 1900's, it is negligible in the so-called primitive countries. Among wild animals, heart trouble is nonexistent.

For our hearts' sake, Americans obviously need to take a few backward steps. We must give up processed foods and cigarettes, but even more important, we must take up physical activity. This combination is the secret of averting heart disease. This secret will help more than one reader to double his lifespan. A potential heart-attack victim who would probably drop dead in his forties may instead live on to his eighties or beyond, by following the correct living habits.

This health and longevity secret has been taken advantage of by a knowledgeable few for some time. They combine exercise with the avoidance of cigarettes, refined foods, and animal fats. As might be expected, these individuals build and maintain heart and circulatory systems nearly immune to disorder.

Of course, the success of a few individuals does not provide conclusive proof, but this theory is also being proved with large groups. Here and there a progressive doctor or physical trainer sponsors adult males (the class most vulnerable to heart trouble) in a program like the one I have just described.

One of these pioneers is Dr. Thomas K. Cureton, director of the Physical Fitness Research Laboratory of the

University of Illinois. Dr. Cureton has trained and tested more than ten thousand middle-aged men. *Time* magazine quotes him as saying: "I can't find one man who followed my plan diligently, who ever suffered a heart attack."

If the average American is lucky enough to avoid heart disease, the next greatest health threat is cancer. Nearly one million Americans are being treated for cancer, and more than three hundred and fifty thousand die each year. As a destroyer of life, cancer is second only to heart ailments. In the United States, it now accounts for about 20% of all deaths; yet, cancer is unknown among groups who live naturally.

Dr. Price, in his studies of primitive peoples throughout the world, found that cancer, like heart disease, was nonexistent. Dr. McCarrison, in nine years of living among the Hunzans and treating their minor ailments, failed to observe a single case of cancer.

In earlier days, cancer must also have been nonexistent. In postmortem examinations of thirty thousand mummified bodies of ancient Egyptians, not one showed signs of cancer. What a contrast to the United States in the twentieth century! Our cancer rate is higher than that of any country in history. It is now estimated that, at some time in life, one out of three Americans will develop this dread disease.

Cancer, like heart trouble, is obviously a disease of modern civilization, and it also began its unwelcome rise in the early 1900's. The basic causes of both heart trouble and cancer are usually much the same. As with heart trouble, the development of cancer appears to be connected with a refined diet, cigarette smoking, and other banes of our modern age, and though it is probably a lesser factor than in cases of heart trouble, lack of exercise also seems to play a part.

In an earlier chapter, I discussed the relationship between cancer and an insufficient supply of oxygen to the body's cells. The best way to flood the cells with oxygen is through exercise. During heightened activity, the cells receive two to two and a half times as much oxygen as usual, so it would seem that exercise might be a useful weapon for combating cancer.

That this may be so has been indicated by research on animals. In an experiment conducted at Jefferson Medical College in Philadelphia, cancer was transplanted into the bodies of rats. Some of the animals were forced to remain inactive by being confined to small individual cages, others were forced to indulge in strenuous daily exercise, such as running for many miles or swimming for hours.

The cancers in the unexercised rats grew to from five to ten times the weight of those in the overexercised group. Among the exercising rats, the cancer growth was not only inhibited, but in some cases the cancer disappeared completely.

More research appears to be in order in this field. Perhaps exercise, along with other natural means, might prove to be as effective a deterrent to cancer, as it is to heart disease.

As for other diseases, there is evidence which indicates that their presence can also be affected by exercise. Arthritis, diabetes, multiple sclerosis, emphysema, ulcers, osteoporosis, varicose veins, and other ailments have favorably responded to exercises. This form of therapy may also prove effective in their prevention as well.

It would seem quite possible for exercise to be found to be a potent factor in the treatment and prevention of disease. As *Clinical Nutrition* editor, Jean Mayer, Ph.D., observes: "It may well be that no currently available medical measure could be as beneficial as an increase in the amount of exercise taken by our population." [1]

---

[1] *Clinical Nutrition*, December, 1966.

One reason I place exercise at the top of the list of health and longevity aids is that it can, to a great extent, make amends for neglect of other factors.

Many observers have noticed that most of those who are healthy and long-lived eat the same foods as the rest of the populace; however, these healthy oldsters almost invariably led lives filled with physical activity.

In his health magazine, *The Provoker*, editor John Tobe, a champion of health through proper diet, also pays tribute to exercise: "Anyone who has read any amount of my writings will no doubt have learned that I have stressed the value of proper diet in health. In fact, I have for some years pressed its importance more than any other single fact or principle. And while I will not back down on my firm conviction and belief, I also must accept the truth that physical labor or exercise is equally important in the prevention of most physical impairments and diseases.

"The reason I am compelled to add this corollary is because I have through my lifetime known hundreds, yes absolutely hundreds, of men and women who violated practically every biological law and yet they remained in comparatively good health and lived to a normal or ripe old age. But in every one of these cases the party involved indulged in strenuous exercise or hard labor all his life."

Exercise can, to some extent, also make up for violation of still another important health and longevity principle: maintaining a tranquil mind. The person who, by temperament or misfortune, is subject to mental stress can lighten or even eliminate his emotional stress by means of muscular exertion.

"Although generalizations are dangerous, I venture to say that at the bottom of many fears, both mild and severe, will be found an overactive mind and an underactive body," writes psychologist Henry C. Link, Ph.D., in *Reader's Digest*. "Hence, I have advised many people, in their quest for happiness, to use their heads less and their arms and legs more—in useful work or play. We generate fears while we sit; we overcome them by action. Fear is nature's warning signal to get busy." [2]

SUMMARY

The leading health and longevity factor is physical activity.

[2] Excerpt from "Do the Thing You Fear," Henry C. Link, Ph.D. *Reader's Digest*, December 1937. Used by permission.

thirty

Euphoria

By now you may be asking what kind of activity is best able to guard you against sickness and prolong your life. Lifting heavy weights, or performing tedious calisthenics?

When I first began to investigate exercise as a good-health, long-life factor, specific information was hard to find. After much search, study, and thought, I reached the conclusion that exercise, to be of most benefit, must be frequent, vigorous, prolonged, and rhythmic, and that it must make use of the legs.

You don't have to struggle with ponderous weights or practice monotonous calisthenics, for these conditions can all be fulfilled by a very simple form of activity. All you need to do to get the boundless benefits exercise offers is to *walk*. If I could give you but one secret of good health and long life, it would be *walk*. Never pass up a chance to walk. Instead of riding to the store, walk. Instead of taking an elevator, walk up and down stairs. Instead of watching a half-hour television show, take a brisk half-hour walk. Instead of riding to and from work, walk. Walk every day, if possible, and the farther, the better.

There is a wonderful world all around us that most people miss completely. This world is seen only by the walker. Exploring it will heighten the pleasure walking brings you.

The walker sees so much that the motorist misses. After riding on a road in an automobile, I am always surprised at how much more I see by walking along the same route. In a car, you go *through* territory, but on foot, you are a *part* of that territory.

On a country road, many sights that you didn't previously notice come into clear view: fruit growing on a tree, a moss-covered rock, a bee lighting on a flower, a wriggling garter snake in the road, or a fish in a stream. When walking, it is easy to stop and observe such things of interest. It is also easy to stop and enjoy the many beautiful views you'll encounter.

Something about nature appeals to all of us. Perhaps our two-million-year heritage of living in the open, surrounded by the wonders and the beauties of the outdoors, has left an indelible mark on us all.

City walking also has its delights. You may think you know your community, but not until you cover it on foot will you see the real city. Then you'll be able to enjoy, at firsthand, the sights and sounds of your city's various neighborhoods, its buildings—"antique," modern, and in between, its shops, and its interesting people.

To gain the utmost benefit from walking, walk at a fast pace. The faster you walk, the more health benefits you will gain. In addition, walking rapidly is a time-saver, for you derive more good in less time. However, in the beginning, you must want to walk at a relatively slow pace, and then work up to a faster rate as you become accustomed to using your legs.

To attain the extra health and longevity that you can get from physical activity, all you ever need do is walk.

But after you have begun to feel the excellent effects you have gained by the simple act of walking, you may decide to advance to an even more beneficial form of leg work. When you have worked up to walking fast, you may feel ready for a slightly more vigorous activity, which will, of course, be even more beneficial to your heart and to the rest of your system.

To learn which forms of exercise provide the most health benefits, Major Kenneth H. Cooper conducted tests on thousands of U.S. airmen. He discovered that three types of exercise were even superior to walking. Major Cooper rated as the most beneficial forms of exercise, running, swimming, bicycling, and walking, in that order.

Whichever method of exercise you adopt—walking, biking, swimming, or running—it will bring you incalculable health returns. If you wish, you can, of course, practice more than one form of activity. Running is my mainstay, but I also walk and bicycle. I run for my life, but I hike and bike primarily for enjoyment.

If you are pressed for time to exercise, slow running requires the least time in ratio to benefits you will gain from it. Fifteen minutes of slow running will bring you as much benefit or more as, for example, one hour of fast walking.

A relatively slow rate of running is all that is needed to gain top health benefits. You don't need to match the record of a young athlete. The pace that is fast enough to make you puff is the one that will help you to health.

For those who can't manage continuous running, or who are at the intermediate stage of progress between walking to running, alternate running and walking is a good practice.

One thing about increasing your physical activity may be bothering you. "Isn't vigorous exercise tiring?" you may ask. "I'm already tired much of the time. Where will I get the energy to exercise?" You will get it by exercising.

Few people realize that vigorous exercise seems to create energy, rather than use it up. When the tired business man returns from work, he only wants to rest, but a better antidote for his tiredness would be exercise.

"To many experiencing a good workout at this time of day, it seems a miracle that fatigue should disappear and energy emerge so quickly," says *Exercising for Physical Fitness*, a booklet issued by the President's Council on Physical Fitness. "Actually it is quite simple. During exercise, as the circulatory and respiratory systems are stimulated and the blood begins to surge through the body, oxygen and nutrients are fed to the cells of the tissues and the accumulated waste products are removed."

The renewal of energy by means of exercise was noted by Dr. Theodore G. Klumpp, a member of an American Medical Association committee that studied the subject of human aging, who wrote in *Prevention* magazine: "The mental and emotional fatigue that comes at the end of a trying but sedentary day can be miraculously dispelled with a little physical exercise. It takes a particular exertion of will to undertake physical activity when fatigue is already present and one's whole being is crying out for rest—or perhaps a drink. But over and over again it has been demonstrated that physical activity in such circumstances brings a degree of refreshment and renewed energy that nothing else can equal." [1]

One of exercise's most pleasant attributes is its effectiveness as a tranquilizer. The tranquilizing effect of exercise begins to make itself felt soon after activity begins. When I walk rapidly, run slowly, or bicycle, I begin to

[1] *Prevention*, November 1970.

feel tensions draining from me within minutes. This is at times almost a physical feeling, as if the tensions were flowing down my body and out through my moving feet.

I must warn you that exercise may prove habit-forming. You may soon find yourself eagerly anticipating this activity. I often discover myself actually craving the feeling of well-being I have learned to expect from my exercise sessions.

Once you discover the joys of using your legs, you may become addicted to physical activity, as many others have. You will then no longer need to be coaxed to get on your feet and use them. You will look forward to each outing with pleasure. Among those I know who exercise regularly —even so little as walking a few blocks a day—not one of them has failed to notice and to comment on the improvement brought about in the way he or she feels.

One of the advantages of slow running over other activity is that it brings on the phenomenal feeling of euphoria most quickly. When you are walking or bicycling, euphoria doesn't usually hit you until hours have elapsed. This sensation can be more quickly achieved through slow running.

Shortly after you become a slow runner, you will begin to experience the sensation of euphoria, that feeling of sheer bliss, exaltation, and extraordinary well-being.

One running enthusiast described his achievement of euphoria: "When I had been running an hour or more a day for about a month, I began to experience a new pleasure. After about five minutes, I felt an increase in energy. My legs seemed to feel as if they just wanted to go bounding and skimming along. My breathing became easy and comfortable and I felt an unusual optimism and confidence. Never in my life had I felt so fully alive!"

Exercising for Physical Fitness has this to say about

running and the feeling of euphoria: "This rejuvenation process in such a short period as thirty to fifty minutes is so dramatic that even after one has enjoyed the resultant state of euphoria a number of times, it still seems unbelievable."

I have experienced the marvelous feeling of euphoria again and again. The first time I felt it was twenty-seven years ago, when as I was pushing my first-born in her stroller on a country road, a wonderful feeling of joy and contentment swept over me. Since then I have enjoyed euphoria many times, most often among the beauties of nature during a hike or bike ride with one or more members of my family.

SUMMARY

The most beneficial forms of exercise are running, swimming, bicycling, and walking.

thirty-one

Good Things Happen

When you indulge in vigorous physical activity regularly, many good things happen inside your body. Amazing physical changes take place in your heart and in your circulatory system. Some of these are:

1. *Exercise reduces cholesterol in the blood vessels.* Cholesterol is the harmful substance which tends to clog arteries and veins. Many studies show that blood cholesterol levels are lower in those who exercise than in those who don't.

2. *The arteries grow larger.* Arteries are as much as four or five times larger in those who exercise regularly and vigorously. When arteries are larger in size, the chances of their being blocked by cholesterol are greatly reduced.

3. *Exercise increases the number of capillaries.* Capillaries are tiny blood vessels, through the thin walls of which your cells absorb food and oxygen directly and

return carbon dioxide and other wastes. The more capillaries you have the more channels you have for receiving nutrients and removing wastes. In guinea pigs that were encouraged to exercise vigorously, the capillaries in certain muscle tissue increased 40 to 45%.

4. *Exercise creates extra blood.* With more blood, you increase your capacity to carry nourishment to cells and remove waste from them. Tests show that regular, vigorous exercise can increase blood volume by nearly a full quart.

5. *Exercise reduces blood pressure.* High blood pressure is often a forerunner to heart disease. Before-and-after checks show that regular exercise usually lowers blood pressure.

6. *The resting pulse rate is lowered.* Dr. Raymond Pearl's research proved that those with a slower pulse rate lived longer. Many other studies have confirmed these findings. For example, insurance company statisticians have learned that in people with pulse rates of 90 to 100, the number of cancer deaths is about 60% higher than average.

The explanation of how regular exercise reduces pulse rate is simple. The heart muscle becomes stronger and more efficient with training, and it pumps more blood with each beat. Therefore, it does not need to beat as often; consequently, when at rest, the heart of the habitual exerciser pumps at a slower rate.

One study of Olympic athletes revealed the effects of various athletic activities on the pulse, ranging from those activities which required no endurance to those which required a great deal. Average pulse rates were: weight lifters—80; sprinters—65; long-distance cyclists—64½; middle-distance runners—63; long-distance runners—61; and marathon runners—58.

The normal pulse rate is 72, but instead of being truly

"normal," this rate actually is the *average* rate. A truly normal pulse rate would be much lower, for it would be the rate of the well-exercised minority, in the 50's or low 60's.

Some marathon runners and milers have attained fantastically low pulse rates. The lowest that I have found on record are: Paavo Nurmi and Roger Bannister—38; Les MacMitchell—32; Bill Dodson—30.

I hope I haven't frightened you with this discussion of distance running. You don't have to run 26-mile marathons to develop a low pulse rate, for you can actually do this with surprisingly little effort. My pulse rate, for example, was substantially lowered by running an average of only a few minutes a day.

Before I fully appreciated the possible benefits to be gained, I ran only on a hit-or-miss basis. Some days I did more, other days less; on many days nothing. My efforts averaged perhaps ten minutes a day three or four times a week. After a number of years on this limited program, I first read of Dr. Pearl's findings regarding pulse rate. Naturally I wondered what effect, if any, my activities had had on my pulse rate. I hoped that, in spite of the meagerness of my exercise program, I had brought my pulse down to at least a little below the so-called normal, 72. I was, therefore, astonished to discover that my pulse rate was down to around 50, varying between 47 to 52. Since I have increased my exercise, I have achieved a still lower pulse, and my new low is now 43.

From this, you can see that long-distance running is not necessary to bring about a substantial reduction in pulse rate. Many who take up running reduce their pulse rate to around 50 within a few months.

The best time to check your pulse rate is upon awakening in the morning, before you get up. At that time, the rate is not affected by any of the various conditions that can cause the heart to beat faster, such as eating, drinking, taking stimulants, smoking, standing, heat, activity, and many other factors.

The normal pulse rate for women is slightly higher than it is for men. The rate for growing children varies, but it is much higher than that of adults.

In some elderly people who do not exercise, the pulse rate has slowed down, but this is the result of impaired heart rhythm.

One more thing about checking your pulse: If you are inclined to be high-strung, concentration on your pulse may cause it to speed up. Once you get accustomed to taking your pulse, however, you will learn your true pulse rate.

Doesn't strenuous exercise result in an enlarged heart? It certainly does. The more the heart, or any muscle, is exercised, the bigger and stronger it becomes. The heart will respond to the demands put on it by exercise by growing larger and stronger, just as the biceps muscle of your arm would enlarge and strengthen if you regularly practice chinning exercises.

X-rays of the hearts of the athletes who participated in the 1928 Olympic games showed that distance runners had the largest hearts. Second were the oarsmen and long-distance bicycle riders, whose hearts were almost as large as those of the distance runners. Middle distance runners had somewhat smaller hearts. The hearts of the sprinters were smaller still, being not much bigger than those of the general population.

The same kind of ratio holds true for animals. The heart of the lean race horse is larger than that of the husky work horse. Birds which fly have larger hearts than ground birds like chickens. The creature that has the largest heart in proportion to its weight is the hummingbird, whose wings beat so fast that the movement is not visible to the naked eye.

The heart which has been enlarged by strenuous activity is actually the one which should be considered normal. The so-called normal hearts of the underexercised are really abnormal, and those who know about exercise and the heart call them "loafer's hearts" or "civilized hearts."

The enlarged heart of the type sometimes found in heart disease is a different type of enlargement, for it is a dilation caused by weakness of the heart muscle.

You may be wondering about the fellow with a bad heart. Surely, he must avoid anything but the mildest exertion, because the least strenuous activity might aggravate his condition. This was once the accepted viewpoint, even among doctors. Only a few years ago, a heart attack meant weeks or months of rigid bed rest for the patient, and activity thereafter was strictly limited. As recently as 1956, a medical textbook advised restricting a heart-patient's activity to "walking short distances on level ground and playing croquet."

But this kind of thinking is being replaced by the theory that exercise taken early and often will speed recovery. According to Dr. Louis F. Bishop, past president of the American College of Cardiology: "There is no cardiovascular condition where some form of exercise is not helpful."

This new formula for recovery is being validated by use on actual heart-disease patients. Many heart-disease sufferers now take the treatments prescribed by Dr. Cureton and other practitioners who believe in exercise.

Bill Cumler, director of businessmen's programs of the Cleveland YMCA, has acquired a national reputation as a result of his work with heart cases. Many of Cumler's "patients" are heart-attack victims. He starts them on the light activity of walking in waist-deep water. They then progress to walking and jogging on a track, and eventually, some run as far as ten miles at a time.

Dr. Carleton B. Chapman, past president of the American Heart Association, also treats heart patients by the use of physical activity. Once a patient can get out of bed, Dr. Chapman puts him on a program of exercise, which begins with walking a mile or two a day. In time, many of Dr. Chapman's heart cases progress to walking, bicycling, or running four or five miles daily. (Dr. Chapman himself runs five miles every morning.) If you suffer from a heart condition, you should only exercise under the supervision of a doctor or a physical instructor who is versed in exercise therapy.

Another good reason for ranking physical activity above the other health and longevity factors is its power to lessen the harmful effects of emotional turmoil.

Mental tension is worked off through exercise, and its harmful effects are minimized. Instead of building up, nervous pressures are dissipated.

That exercise can nullify the harmful effects of emotional agitation has been proved in the experiments conducted by Dr. Hans Selye, who is recognized as the world's leading authority on stress. Today's stress-filled life is often defined as a rat race. Appropriately, Dr. Selye first conducted his experiments with rats. This is the account of these experiments reported in *Reader's Digest*: "Selye took ten sedentary laboratory rats, stressed them with shocks, blinding lights, ear-splitting noises, and pain. Within a month, every rat was dead. Using a treadmill, Dr. Selye then trained ten more rats, same age and breed, until they were conditioned like human distance runners. Then he applied the same stresses. After a month of stress, the conditioned rats were well and thriving! Repeating the experiment, he found that untrained rats died, trained rats lived. The lesson: exercise trains the nerves to resist stress. The eminent scientist is today a strong advocate of physical fitness." [1]

Remember this story of the exercising rats and what it shows. By practicing regular, vigorous leg work you may also cancel the damage caused by life's inevitable stresses. Like Selye's distance-running rats, you too can run away from the health-destroying, life-shortening effects of emotional stress.

SUMMARY

Regular, vigorous physical activity creates many beneficial physical changes within your body, which help counteract the harmful effects of emotional stress.

[1] *Reader's Digest*, July 1965.

thirty-two

Where, When, and How

I have already told you *why* you should exercise. I will now tell you where, when, how, and how much.

Where should you exercise? In the best place available. I am now speaking mostly about running, but much of what I say also applies to walking and cycling. Perhaps the most pleasant exercise route is a country path that runs through fields or woods, or a path in a park. But public sidewalks also make good running tracks, if you don't mind a few curious stares. The best time for running on city sidewalks is around 6 P.M., during the dinner hour, when the fewest number of people are abroad.

If no sidewalks are handy, you may have to run in the road. If you must use a road or highway, find one that has little vehicular traffic, and stay on the correct side of it. According to law, pedestrians—and this includes runners as well as walkers—must keep to the left, to face oncoming traffic. Cyclists, however, are considered part of the traffic, and they must keep to the right.

The ideal surface on which to run is, of course, a running track. Most cities, even smaller ones, have at least one athletic field that has a measured track, and this may be available to you for your workouts. Most of the time this track will not be in use, so it's almost like having your own private track. If you are the fortunate owner of an acre or so of land, you can truly have your own running path. Even a large back yard can accommodate a suitable path.

If you prefer exercising in strict privacy, you can walk or run as far as you desire without leaving your home. Just step on the movable platform of an exercise machine, and away you go. You can walk or run as far as you wish, without going anywhere. If you find stationary indoor exercise boring, you can walk or run to the accompaniment of radio or television. Walker-runner machines are advertised in health magazines.

It is nice to have one of these machines in the winter, when snow, ice, and frigid temperatures make outdoor exercise difficult. After fifteen years of struggling through snow and slush every winter and sometimes having frozen fingers and toes, I finally bought a walker-runner. I now run all winter in comfort. However, my wintertime arrangement is only a temporary expedient. Each winter, I can hardly wait for spring to arrive so I can get back outside, under the sky, with the fields and woods stretching out around me.

Some people run at home without using a machine. They simply run in place, lifting the feet off the floor as if running.

Get all the oxygen you can if you exercise indoors. Work out near an open window.

Another way of exercising while dodging curious stares or wintry weather is by running around the perimeter of a gymnasium. You may not get so much fresh air as you would like in a gym, for many gyms are poorly ventilated. But this isn't nearly as important as getting the exercise.

Some smart exercisers kill two birds with one stone by walking, bicycling, or running to and from work.

When should you exercise? Whenever you prefer, or whenever it is most convenient. Some people like to work out in the morning before breakfast, when energy is at a peak, but many prefer the end of the day, when energy is lower. Exercise brings a welcome energy pick-up at this time of day.

Exercise whenever you please, but the important thing is to do it regularly.

In the beginning, be careful of overdoing. You may end up with sore muscles, or worse. Unless you are already in condition from some other activity, your muscles, including your heart, probably aren't ready for vigorous exercise.

To be on the safe side, you could start with short walks, gradually increasing speed and distance, walking a little faster and a bit farther each day. Finally, you could switch to very slow running, gradually increasing speed and distance again.

Exercise regularly. Follow your routine daily if possible. Skip few, if any, exercise periods. On some days, you may feel like doing a bit more, on other days, a bit less. However, you should try hard to maintain a daily schedule. It is the *regular* exerciser who benefits, and the weekend athlete who risks unfavorable reactions.

Always precede your exercise session with a short warm-up period. Athletes, some of whom learned the hard way, know that to avoid a pulled muscle or an even more serious injury, muscles must be warmed up before they undergo heavy exertion. Before getting down to the serious business of competition, the runner jogs, the football player does calisthenics, and the weight-lifter raises light weights. You should also begin to exercise by running or bicycling at a very slow pace before tackling faster movements.

Taper off gradually after exercise. Just as you warmed up, you must cool down. Walk around for a few minutes after running or bicycling. This action will continue to pump the leg veins, and it will help your heart adjust to the easing off of activity.

If it becomes necessary to lay off exercising for any length of time for any reason, start with relatively light activity when you begin again, and increase your speed and distance a little each day.

Don't exercise beyond your capacity. Extremely strenuous exercise is never necessary. You can achieve good results without pushing yourself too far. Never compete with anyone, or against the clock, for this may be a temptation to overdo.

Don't indulge in strenuous exercise too soon after eating. Allow yourself at least three hours to digest your food; otherwise, your muscles will rob blood from your digestive system, which is where it is needed.

Curtail heavy activity during extreme weather. Exercising in extreme heat can bring on heat stroke. Reduce your activity during hot weather, or avoid the heat by scheduling your workout for either early or late in the day.

During very cold weather, exercise indoors, because extreme cold places an added burden on the heart. A weak heart may be adversely affected by exercising in excessive cold.

Don't go to bed right after exercising, for you may be too keyed up to sleep. Give your system at least an hour to return to normal before retiring.

Low oxford-type shoes are best for running. Sneakers or low-cut soft-soled canvas shoes are the most comfortable. If you discover the tendency to develop foot blisters when walking or running, wear two pairs of socks. Wear thin cotton socks next to the feet, with a heavier woolen pair over them. This cuts down the friction between the shoes and feet.

Dogs are an annoyance frequently encountered by the exerciser, especially in the country. Most dogs are friendly, and running up to a stranger and barking is their way to express friendliness. But if you find dogs annoying, there's a simple way to send them away. Down through the centuries, the dog has acquired a fear of the man with a stone. You don't have to carry stones around to get rid of dogs, however. Instead, when a dog bothers you, simply bend over, pick up an imaginary stone, and pretend to throw it at him. I have never known these gestures to fail to make a dog retreat.

Some exercisers are lone wolves who prefer to work out by themselves. Others are more gregarious and enjoy company. If you would prefer one or more exercising partners, consult your local Y.M.C.A., where you can get in touch with interested parties, or perhaps join an already-active group. Some people have located exercising partners by placing an ad in the newspaper.

In the past, athletes were told not to drink water during exercise. This may have been because drinking water while exercising causes slight nausea in a few people. But it is now thought that, even in the midst of exercise, thirst should be satisfied. During prolonged strenuous exertion, the body loses water through perspiration and through the lungs, and unless this water is replaced, dehydration can occur.

During exercise, substances other than water are lost and will later need to be replaced. One of the substances is salt.

Some authorities recommend that extra salt intake accompany each period of heavy perspiration. Others insist that ordinary salt is harmful, and that, under any circumstances, the healthful natural salt in foods is all that the body needs. The latter group advises instead an increased intake of Vitamin C. Analysis of perspiration reveals the presence of considerable Vitamin C. Coal miners who perspire heavily sometimes develop scurvy in spite of what would otherwise be a sufficient intake of Vitamin C.

One expert, N. N. Yakovlev, of the Academy of Sciences in Russia, places the need for Vitamin C of the competitive endurance athlete at four times the regular requirement. Even though your efforts are noncompetitive, you would be wise to maintain a high Vitamin C intake.

Other nutrients which need extra replenishment after exercise are the B Vitamins and the minerals sodium, potassium, and calcium. The vigorous exerciser would, therefore, do well to maintain a high consumption of citrus fruit (for Vitamin C), brewer's yeast or liver (for the B Vitamins), and kelp (for all minerals).

Here are a few precautions to observe in connection with the preceding advice on how to exercise.

If any untoward symptoms develop, stop exercising at once. If you feel faint or dizzy, if your heart pounds excessively, if you experience trouble in breathing, if you feel pain, or if you feel excessively tired, stop.

If you suffer from a heart condition or some other ailment, are overweight, are dieting, or are anemic, don't take up exercise without a doctor's approval, and then do so only under his supervision.

Check with your doctor after any illness before resuming your program. If he approves, resume your exercise gradually.

Don't try to treat an ailment by exercising. Check with your doctor, and if he approves exercise as a treatment, carry it out under his supervision.

Even a moderate amount of regular exercise is enough to bring incalculable benefit, but for most substantial health rewards, I recommend that you gradually work up to one of the following daily activities: (1) a half hour of slow running or swimming, (2) two hours of fast walking, (3) one hour of fairly fast bicycling, or (4) a combination of any two, or all three of these.

One of these activities should constitute your *minimum* daily activity. If you eventually choose to progress further, so much the better.

In recommending plenty of exercise, I don't just preach it, I also do it. This advice comes from a person who has frequently for many years used his legs, vigorously and protractedly. I have been running—although on a limited scale at first—for nearly twenty years.

It took a little courage for me to take up running when I was nearly forty years old, back in the early 1950's. At that time the prevalent notion was that strenuous activity would damage the heart. But I was beginning to see that physical activity had more than a little to do with all health, including the health of the heart. I am still here, and I am still running. I have lived to see exercise become recognized as a means of protecting the health of the heart.

Today, my usual daily run is about five miles, and it takes almost three-quarters of an hour. On the occasional day when I am low on pep, I sometimes do less than five miles; when I have extra energy, I run faster or farther, or both. On a particularly good day, I have run as far as thirteen miles. I run almost every day, rain or shine, winter or summer.

In company with other exercise enthusiasts, I feel better when I do more, not less, exercise. In addition to running, I frequently hike or bike in the country, mainly for enjoyment, but the accompanying health benefits are most welcome.

I have been addressing myself to the men in my audience, but what I have said also applies for the most part to the women and children. It is safe to say that most women and a great many children are underexercised today.

Women, like men, have a built-in need for exercise. For two million years, women took part in strenuous activity. Although their tasks were less arduous than men's, they were far from light. Women did not hunt, but they contributed to the food supply by gathering wild fruits and vegetables. When people began to wear clothes, the women made coarse animal skins into clothing. Later, when people began to farm, it was usually the women who hoed the ground and planted the crops. Women also made pottery, ground grain with large stones, and performed a great variety of other needed tasks. While the men hunted, the women did most of the other work.

Women today don't exert themselves as much as in former days; yet, it must be admitted that most housewives get more exercise than their husbands. Women move about on their legs while performing housework, which is probably another reason they now outlive males, most of whom are more sedentary.

But in this electrical age, housework no longer provides sufficient exercise, even for the smaller muscles of women. With more exertion, women could live still longer.

Some women are starting to learn the value of exercise. One woman who began to take long walks after dinner found that she lost six pounds a week. Another who started to run reported that her energy had increased, that she felt better, and that she had lost thirty pounds. She now says, "My housework may not always get done, but my running does!"

A generation or two ago, children used their legs a great deal. Today, many of them are chauffeured almost everywhere they go, and television often replaces vigorous play. As a result, our children are so appallingly underexercised that a third of them can't pass simple physical-achieve-ment tests. In foreign countries, less than one child in ten fails such tests.

Elderly people need exercise just as much as younger people do—perhaps even more so. From his studies of Russian centenarians, longevity expert Professor A. Nagorny concludes: "It should be considered as proved that one of the necessary conditions of longevity is constant, and sometimes quite tense work, very often continuing almost right up until death."

Marathon runners have proved that strenuous endurance activity can be continued in later years. These athletes last longer than any others. Some marathon runners continue to compete when in their fifties and sixties.

Many older men keep in good condition by exercising regularly and vigorously. *Strength and Health* magazine-publisher Bob Hoffman took up running when well past middle age. A few years ago, he celebrated his sixty-ninth birthday by running fifteen miles, breaking his distance record. Bernard Baruch, the noted financier, was a physical-activity enthusiast. He swam three or four times a week until his death at age ninety-four.

Amos Alonzo Stagg, the famous football coach, still trained with his teams when he was in his eighties, regularly practiced running until he was ninety-six, coached until he was ninety-eight, and lived to be one hundred and two.

The value of activity for the elderly was demonstrated by careful before and after tests in one exercise experiment. Forty-one men between the ages of fifty and eighty-seven were put through a program of jogging and other exercise by Herbert A. DeVries, a physical education professor at the University of Southern California. According to his tests, in only six weeks' training, DeVries' elderly exercisers lost 4.9% of their body fat, reduced blood pressure 6%, raised their oxygen-consuming ability by 9.2%, and reduced nervous tension 15%.

DeVries' conclusions, according to *Time*, were that "exercise makes the bodies of septuagenarians act like those of forty-year-olds."

The best advice I can give you for health and longevity is this: Man or woman, young or old, get off your seat and onto your feet.

Summary

To exercise, begin with light activity and gradually increase speed and distance each day. Exercise daily or almost daily. Always precede vigorous exercise with a light warm-up, and finish by tapering off gradually. After a lay-off, begin again with relatively light activity and increase speed and distance each day. Don't indulge in strenuous activity until at least three hours after eating, and don't exercise beyond your capacity. Curtail heavy activity during weather extremes. Replace nutrients lost in exercising.

If any untoward symptoms develop, stop at once. If you suffer from a heart condition or other ailment, are overweight, dieting, anemic, or over forty, don't take up exercise without your doctor's approval, and then only under his supervision. Check with your doctor after any illness before resuming your program, and don't try to treat an ailment by exercising on your own.

For substantial health rewards, work up to a half hour of slow running or swimming, two hours of fast walking, one hour of fast bicycling, or a combination of any two or all three.

One of the above should constitute your *minimum* daily activity. If you eventually choose to progress further, so much the better.

thirty-three

Take It Off

Statistics compiled by insurance companies prove that those who are overweight die younger. Fat people are more susceptible to heart disease, diabetes, and other ailments.

I will discuss being overweight only briefly, for it should pose no great problem to the conscientious follower of the health system I advocate. If you are of normal weight, my program should automatically keep you that way. If you are overweight at the start of the program, it should help you to reduce and stay reduced.

Being overweight is a dangerous condition which is the result of a combination of too much food and not enough exercise. The body stores the food not burned for energy for future use. It is saved, in the form of fat, for a rainy day, but for those who become obese, this rainy day never comes.

The foods responsible for obesity are the energy foods, carbohydrates and fats. If you take in more of these foods than you burn up, you gain weight, but if your body burns these energy producers about as fast as you take them in, your body weight remains the same. If you burn more than you take in, you lose weight.

The "carbos" most conducive to gaining weight are those that have been refined and cooked. These foods are more easily and rapidly digested than the natural, raw kind. A meal heavy in refined, cooked carbos overwhelms the body with more carbohydrate than it can use. Some of the excess calories then become stored fat.

But even whole and wholesome foods can cause you to become overweight if you consume them to excess, especially if they aren't being used up by activity. If you find that you remain overweight in spite of frequent, lengthy exercise sessions, you need to cut down on carbohydrates and fats.

Among the foods those who are overweight should eat in moderation are carbohydrates such as bread—even the whole-grain kind, dried peas, beans, and lentils; dried figs, dates, raisins, and prunes; honey, molasses, and maple sugar. Although they are whole and nutritious, these foods are still carbohydrates and are capable of adding unwanted pounds.

Also high in obesity-producing calories are fats, such as butter, oil, fatty meat, nuts, and peanuts.

Some words of warning to over-enthusiastic dieters are in order here. Many reducers suffer irreparable health damage from reducing diets that are one-sided. A reducing diet should be short in carbohydrates and fats, but it must not exclude vital proteins, minerals, and vitamins. While cutting down on the fats and carbohydrates the weight-reducer should maintain a sufficient intake of protein foods, and a high intake of vitamin and mineral foods.

Moreover, carbohydrates and fats should not be completely eliminated. They are vital elements that are necessary to health and life, and no one can get along without them. No diet, not even one to reduce weight, should be entirely devoid of fats and carbohydrates, so the weight-watcher must be sure that his diet contains at least a little of these necessary substances.

Some fat people eat lightly at meal times, and yet they remain overweight. They keep their weight up by nibbling between meals. Cheating with between-meal snacks (except for raw fruits and vegetables, or their juices) can defeat the best reducing diet.

Alcohol, though not in itself fattening, does contribute to the formation of body fat. Even when a low-carbohydrate, low-fat diet is strictly adhered to, the fat person may find it hard to lose weight if he continues to consume alcoholic beverages. Both food and alcohol contribute calories, but there is a difference between food calories and alcohol calories. Before entering the bloodstream, where they will be put to work furnishing the energy requirements of the body, food calories must first undergo digestion; however, the calories in alcohol enter the bloodstream almost at once. Therefore, the body uses the alcoholic calories first, and stores unneeded food calories as fat, and alcohol replaces food as a source of energy. In this way, alcohol indirectly helps cause overweight, because 95% of the alcohol a person drinks is utilized by the body for energy. The drinker on a low-carbohydrate low-fat regime may, therefore, still fail to lose weight.

A weight-reducing cycle is created by eating less, for as you eat less, your stomach gradually shrinks. As it decreases in size, its demands for food lessen. If you cooperate by continuing your reduced intake, you can get your stomach permanently down to a smaller size, and the rest of you too.

Those who have been overweight often find that it becomes easier to keep to a reducing diet after a fast. During a fast, the stomach shrinks, and afterwards, the appetite is satisfied with less food. Paradoxically, the underweight can also be helped to gain weight by fasting. After a fast, the too-thin may find themselves putting on the pounds they need because freed of its load of toxins, the body is better able to convert food into flesh.

In reducing, the partner of diet is exercise. Exercise burns away calories, whether they are in the form of stored fat or are fresh from food you have only recently eaten.

Exercise can compensate for the lack of will power. The person who indulges in strenuous, prolonged exercise can get away with a heavier calorie consumption without gaining weight. A study of the diets of Olympic athletes, who are, of course, noted for remaining trim, revealed that their daily caloric intake was half again that of the average American. Their regular vigorous training kept these athletes from getting fat.

If you are overweight, it is the result of a combination of too much fattening food and too little exercise. Too many calories and not enough exercise puts pounds on, the opposite takes them off. One thing more is required: patience. It took time to put the weight on, and it will take time to get it off.

As you grow older, it may take a little extra exertion to use up the calories you take in. You may burn fewer calories due to a slowing of your metabolism.

In a few cases, being overweight is the result of a deep-seated metabolic or glandular disorder. People with this condition should not try too hard to reduce; they should forget about weight and just try for good health.

But for most of us, the combination of under-eating and exercise can prevent our being overweight. If we exercise enough, we can even consume more carbohydrates and fats than sedentary persons and still remain trim.

To check on your weight, don't rely on the combination of scales and height-weight tables, which are not reliable guides to proper weight. The correct weight for one person may be the equivalent of overweight or underweight for another. Big bones weigh more than small bones, and muscle tissue weighs more than fat tissue.

Let your mirror be your guide. If any part of your body looks fat, it is time to cut down on calories and step up activity.

Summary

Let your mirror tell you whether you are overweight.

To reduce weight, cut down on carbohydrates and fat foods, but don't cut them out entirely, and exercise.

thirty-four

The Bare-Skin Rug

Each of your body's twenty trillion cells somehow knows what its job is and how to do it. A muscle cell does what a muscle cell should do, a liver cell behaves like a liver cell, and a bone cell does the tasks a bone cell must do.

In performing their functions, cells produce waste. Added to this waste are the bodies of cells which were born, did their job, and died. All these clinkers need to be expelled. This is the job of the bloodstream. The same bloodstream that carries food and oxygen to your cells also picks up cell waste and dead cells and carries them to points of elimination. If the constant process of cell purification were halted for even a few hours, you would die, for your cells would drown in their own waste.

Your body's never-ending battle for cell purification will be boundlessly benefited by the program I advocate. Strenuous physical activity, in particular, and most of the other factors as well, will help keep all your eliminative machinery operating efficiently. As long as you follow your health and longevity program faithfully, you will probably be able to forget about your circulatory system and your channels of elimination. They should take good care of their jobs and of themselves automatically. Your four avenues of elimination are the bowels, the kidneys, the lungs, and the skin. The skin is the organ I will discuss next, because I think its eliminative abilities are generally underrated.

Among the eliminative organs, your skin is the largest. If peeled off you in one piece and spread out on the floor, your skin would cover about eighteen square feet. You'd make quite a bare-skin rug.

Some authorities consider the skin of secondary importance to the other channels of elimination. At least one expert does not even consider it an organ of elimination. But the skin, or to be more precise, the skin's 2,500,000 sweat glands, can be an important and valuable part of the eliminative system.

The primary function of the sweat glands is the dissipation of excess body heat. To this end, the composition of perspiration is 98 to 99% water, with only a relatively small amount of waste matter.

When there is no need to cool the body, perspiration amounts to only about a pint a day, but when the 2,500,000 sweat glands are stimulated by heat or by strenuous physical exertion, or by both, their output will increase tremendously. Laborers who work hard in hot temperatures have been known to perspire more than five gallons in eight hours. Football players have lost ten pounds in an hour and a half. When sweat output becomes voluminous, the skin is of considerable help to the other eliminative organs. Then the skin becomes a truly important channel of elimination, which substantially eases the work of the other eliminative organs, particularly the kidneys. When perspiration is heavy, it can be clearly observed that the kidneys are relieved of a great part of their eliminative burden. They pass less urine, even though water intake replaces that lost in perspiration. The urine excreted is also lighter in color and is less strong-smelling than normally.

You should perspire often and profusely. Most of your ancestors did. Unless your exercise sessions leave you wringing wet, you are missing out on some health benefits that are rightfully yours. If necessary, dress heavily while exercising to induce copious perspiration. If you still can't work up a good sweat, you can get one from a sauna bath.

You don't need to build a special sauna room like those used in northern European countries. Small, flexible, plastic saunas are sold by some department stores and health-food dealers. These saunas are just large enough to accommodate one person, who sits inside with his head sticking out through an opening in the top. A small electric heater inside the sauna soon makes the occupant dripping wet. I lose a pound or more an hour in my sauna. This procedure is useless for permanent weight reduction, however, since thirst causes quick replacement of the liquid lost.

Follow all the instructions that come with your sauna, including the warnings. Some ailments, such as heart trouble, can be aggravated by high temperatures, and even those in good health could find too long a sauna session harmful instead of beneficial.

A bath or shower cleans only the skin's surface, but if this soap-and-water cleansing is preceded by a thorough sweat bath, your skin will be clean from the inside as well. It is no wonder that a vigorous sweat-producing workout, followed by a bath or shower, makes you feel "high." To feel even higher, and become even cleaner, you should shed some of your dead skin cells.

Of your body's twenty trillion cells, some are skin cells, which live only four or five days. By then, they become a part of the tough, dead outer layer. Meanwhile, new skin cells are constantly forming underneath, and skin is always being shed and replaced.

You can help speed this process. In between your sweat bath and your soap-and-water bath, take a few minutes to unclog your pores by loosening the dead outer layer of your skin. Without using soap, rub the entire surface of your body with a coarse, wet washcloth. Use the coarsest washcloth you can buy. (Some people use a fairly stiff-bristled, wet brush.) Scrub your entire body, using a firm, brisk circular motion. This rubdown will leave your skin looking and feeling all aglow. Your regular soap and water cleansing routine will complete the process and leave you feeling like a million dollars.

SUMMARY

To help your skin help the other eliminative organs, induce copious perspiration frequently by vigorous exercise or by taking a sauna bath, and help your skin to shed dead cells by rubbing the body with a coarse, wet washcloth or a fairly stiff-bristled, wet brush, then bathe or shower.

thirty-five

The Health Belt

Are some parts of the United States more healthful than others? Is there something about certain areas which makes them conducive to better health and longer life? Various Chambers of Commerce claim that there is, but what do unprejudiced observers say?

Figures released by the National Center for Chronic Disease Control indicate that the longest-lived Americans reside in the central part of the country, in the area that extends from Minnesota to Texas. The Bureau of Census agrees. A map prepared by them that depicts the percentage of population over sixty-five shows a broad longevity belt sweeping down through the center of our nation from Minnesota to Texas.

One small part of this health belt is pinpointed by United States Public Service statistics as being exceptionally favorable to long life. Near the middle of the longevity area, in southeastern Nebraska, lies a cluster of eleven counties in which the average life span is the highest in the nation. The one hundred and thirty-four thousand residents of these eleven Nebraska counties are America's best longevity risks.

Why? Nobody knows. Government experts have considered the possible environmental factors, for perhaps there is something in the air, soil, or drinking water that favors long life. But no proof of such influence has emerged. The only sure fact seems to be that in this eleven-county Nebraska area, people live at least a little longer than anywhere else in the country.

I don't want to sound conceited, but I think I can tell the government experts and you why the people in that Nebraskan Shangri-la live so long. I believe that it is unlikely that their environment contains a youth-preserving elixir. However, a careful analysis of statistics from the health belt does reveal a strong clue as to why the midwest, particularly the eleven-county Nebraska area, is so conducive to longevity. This section of the country is not healthful because of its geographical location but because of something else.

My conclusions as to what *is* responsible for this are borne out by other statistics connected with long life and area of residence. A majority of the long-lived—be they Americans, Hunzans, Russians, or some other nationality —share one common fact about their environment. These people usually live in rural areas, not in big cities.

The biggest proportion of Russian centenarians live in its most rural province, Georgia. The Hunzans live in small villages, and their entire country would hardly make one small city. Dr. Weston Price found his long-lived people in small settlements, and the majority of American oldsters had spent much of their lives in small communities or on farms.

The reason for the midwest's superior longevity record should now be clearer. The vast health belt stretching from Minnesota to Texas is farm country. Big cities are scarce in this area. The entire eleven-county Nebraska longevity tract boasts only one "big" city, Hastings, of which the population is only 21,400.

From all this, it should be obvious that the key geographic factor in longevity is not the *specific part* of the United States in which you live, but what the *size* of your community is.

This view is borne out by a mountain of statistics. Again and again, research has shown that people from rural areas outlive big-city residents. From the stack of statistics I have amassed, I will quote just one, which is typical of them all. Researchers headed by D. M. Berkson learned that deaths from cardiovascular disease in Chicago are twice as common as they are in rural Illinois.

How much longer, on the average, can you expect to live if you make your home in the country rather than in the city? According to a University of Maryland study, five years.

Why is small-town and country living conducive to longevity? What is the connection between rural life and longer life? The reasons can easily be surmised. Early man lived in the wide-open spaces or in small settlements, not in crowded cities. Country and small-town life is more in keeping with the kind of life our earlier ancestors led. Those who live in the country today are more likely to emulate their healthy forebears than are city residents. For example, the country dweller probably enjoys more exposure to sunshine and fresh air. He will also be more likely to use his muscles more often and more vigorously.

Actually, it is not area of residence that is a separate health and longevity factor, but a combination of several factors.

Some of the healthy old-timers in the eleven-county Nebraska area previously discussed were interviewed by a reporter for the *National Enquirer*. A few of their revealing comments follow:

Jim Cutshall, age 101: "Go to bed regular, eat little, and exercise a lot."

Lester Childs, age 96: "I walk a mile a day and always take life with a smile."

Mrs. H. O. Waldo, age 93: "I have loved outdoor work since I picked corn as a girl, and I still love that old garden."

Mrs. Ione Benway, age 93: "I lived on a farm all my life and always did my share of the field work. It's a hard, but healthful life."

W. P. McAdams, age 87: "Hard work is at least part of the answer. I've worked on a farm since I was a kid."

The way of life I advocate can be practiced better in a rural environment than in the city. If you are a city-dweller, moving to the country, if possible, would be to your advantage. But if you are stuck with the city, you can still get most of the health benefits associated with rural life by faithfully following your program of natural living. It's the nearest thing to country living in the city.

SUMMARY

Country or small-town life is more conducive to health and longevity than city living. If you are a city dweller, you can get many of the advantages of country living by following the way of life advocated in this book.

thirty-six

On Borrowed Time

Perhaps, without your knowledge, you are one of the vast army who is living on borrowed time. Millions of Americans are alive today who, were it not for the tremendous strides that have been made in public sanitation, wouldn't be.

Back in the good old days, around 1800, average life expectancy was only about thirty-five years. Today, it is over seventy years. This tremendous upward leap is the result of several factors, the most influential of which is probably public sanitation.

In pre-sanitation days, many virulent diseases were spread by the intestinal discharge of victims and carriers. Improper sewage disposal often contaminated wells or springs, and people who drank from these sources unsuspectingly exposed themselves to deadly disease.

Before we knew that certain infectious diseases were passed along through sewage-contaminated water supplies, ravaging epidemics were common, especially in heavily populated areas. A severe epidemic could destroy a very large portion of a community's population. If the reasons behind these epidemic diseases had not been discovered and proper sanitary precautions had not been instituted and enforced, we would still be oppressed by such population-decimating plagues as those of the past.

Today, many once-feared diseases are all but forgotten.

Typhoid fever, dysentery, and cholera are some of the formerly dreaded killers now subdued by the marvels of public sanitation. Modern government-controlled water supply and sewage disposal systems have eliminated the once common hazard of water-borne disease epidemics.

Additional public-health services, such as pure-food laws and control of disease-bearing insects, also help protect the health and lives of you and your loved ones.

In some backward countries, where sanitary facilities lag or are nonexistent, many people still die who might, under better conditions, survive. For example, in the state of Maranhao in Brazil, life expectancy averages only 29.6 years. In our country, the outlook is far better because of many factors, the most important of which is probably our modern sanitation system.

This country's public-sanitation program is one of the most important influences on your health and longevity. Unlike other good-health, long-life factors from which you benefit mainly through your own efforts, this one comes to you automatically. All you have to do is live in the United States.

Elsewhere in this book, I took the government to task for what I deem to be certain shortcomings in protecting the health and lives of its citizens, but here I want to take the opportunity to doff my hat to Uncle Sam. Thanks to the government's public-sanitation measures, millions now live who otherwise wouldn't.

SUMMARY

One of the most important health and longevity influences is public sanitation. By living in the United States, you enjoy this benefit automatically.

thirty-seven

The Ortho-Docs

The companion of public sanitation in helping mankind is the medical profession. The medical profession has saved the lives of countless numbers. Many who are alive today owe their lives to doctors. Medical science has learned how to forestall, check, or alleviate many of the perils which formerly menaced health and life.

Aided by sanitation, medicine's protective and curative wonders begin in the delivery room, indeed, even before, with prenatal care. Today, the advances in obstetrical care are paying off. In 1915, mothers died during childbirth at the rate of sixty-one per ten thousand live births, but by the time of the 1960 census, this number has dropped to only three. This medical and sanitary protection continues throughout early childhood. In 1915, one baby in ten died before his first birthday. Today this figure has dropped to one in forty.

Medicine's safeguarding activities extend throughout late childhood and adulthood. Vaccination and antibiotics now tame once-dreaded killers, such as polio, rheumatic

226

fever, and other infectious diseases. Surgery, when necessary, mends defects in health brought on by disease or accident.

Despite my strong penchant for avoiding medical treatment, I am the first to acknowledge that there are times when doctors are necessary. The services of medical doctors, when and if needed, can be a highly important factor in regard to your health and longevity.

Notice that I said "when and if needed." You may discover that you have little or no need for doctors after you take out the health insurance expounded in these pages. My health plan is somewhat unorthodox, but it may help you avoid the "ortho-docs."

One kind of medical service which my way of living can help you avoid is a need for surgery. The necessity for surgical removal of any internal organ should be greatly regretted for two reasons: (1) The organ might have been kept sound by proper health habits, and (2) Every bodily organ plays a part in helping to preserve health. Each carries out useful functions, and if at all possible, should remain where nature put it.

Even though some internal organs are not absolutely necessary for survival, they do perform leading roles in fighting infectious diseases. Appurtenances like the tonsils, adenoids, appendix, and thymus—once considered more or less useless vestiges left over from man's evolutionary past—are now being recognized as disease fighters. These bodyguards intercept and confine infectious disease before it can harm vital organs, such as the lungs, liver, or brain.

The function of the tonsils is explained in the *Medical Journal of Australia.* "The exposed position of tonsils and adenoids in the pharynx and their frequent involvement in viral infections lead to the surmise that these tissues have the function to be infected and serve the body by supplying antigens on a physiological level in health, thus maintaining the tonus of the immunological system." [1]

The appendix has also been shown to be an infection fighter. In addition, it appears to be a protection against cancer. Dr. Jay R. McVay, Jr., and Dr. Howard R. Bierman, two researchers who worked independently, have reported that cancer occurs more often in those whose appendix has been removed than in those who have kept this organ.

The thymus gland's importance is demonstrated by the certainty that a baby born without one will soon die of overwhelming infection. Even though the thymus withers in adults, it has been proved to remain an affective health-defender.

The body can struggle along without its tonsils, appendix, or certain other defensive organs, but it will not do as well as it did with them. Lacking some of its defensive equipment, the body is more vulnerable to the serious consequences of infection.

A defensive organ becomes swollen and diseased when it is overworked. Its mighty efforts to survive are evidence of its capability and importance. Cutting out such an organ makes as much sense as firing a policeman because he arrests thieves.

Only in extreme cases—when an organ has deteriorated beyond possibility of healing—should it be removed. Numerous qualified observers, including an increasing number of doctors, believe that many operations are unnecessary and that they, in fact, do more harm than good.

You can help all your organs (as well as the rest of you) stay healthy if you follow the advice in these pages. Although I advocate natural preventive measures against disease and natural methods of self-treatment for minor in-

---

[1] *Medical Journal of Australia*, November 28, 1964.

dispositions, I want to sound a loud warning against amateur medical treatment. If any but the most mild disorder threatens or strikes you, you should be under the care of a doctor. Medical attention may relieve pain, prevent intensification of your ailment, and perhaps even save your life.

SUMMARY

The services of doctors, when and if needed, can be an important health and longevity factor. However, following the advice in these pages may make the need for medical treatment negligible or even totally unnecessary.

thirty-eight

The Malady Lingers On

Regular vigorous physical activity, the maintenance of mental tranquility, a diet containing adequate amounts of the necessary food elements, frequent exposure to sunshine and fresh air, avoiding intake of poisonous substances—these, together with the other natural measures advocated here, are rewarded by good health. Violation of these natural laws is punishable by sickness.

When the average person becomes ill, he is unaware of the fundamental reasons behind his indisposition. If his ailment is of the contagious kind, the victim believes that he "caught" the disease. The sufferer blames a germ, not his incorrect health habits, for his misery.

In truth, the germ didn't actually cause the disease. Disease conditions were already present, brought on by disobedience of nature's laws. Wrong living habits permitted—even encouraged—the accumulation of poisonous waste products. The body was amassing poisons faster than they were being removed. The invading germ was only the spark that set off the flame of disease.

When the *regular* means of elimination fail to cope with mounting waste products, the body sometimes turns to *irregular* means. It resorts to sickness in the form of eliminative illness. In this way, the body seeks to restore its health.

What we call sickness is actually an extraordinary effort of the body to expel an accumulation of toxic substances, or to be more precise, it is the unpleasant symptoms of illness which indicate the body's purification attempt. These symptoms—fever, diarrhea, runny nose, coated tongue, catarrh—are all part of the eliminative process, and although they are unpleasant, they serve the useful purpose of elimination.

Such symptoms are no cause for alarm. Instead, they are a good sign—a sign that the body is conducting a needed clean-up job. Infectious illness, despite its unpleasant symptoms, is not abnormal. Actually, it is the body's healthy reaction to an abnormal condition.

The young and strong body responds most easily to the need for purification. The body not yet weakened by age and decades of wrong living is best capable of intense eliminative action. Fever is most common in the young, rarest in the elderly. Colds, with their many eliminative symptoms, occur most often in those under thirty, least often in those over fifty.

Various hidden causes lie behind the common cold in addition to the cold virus that is the final triggering mechanism. Overeating of starch, too much salt, and even wholesome foods when taken in excess, emotional turmoil, insufficient sleep, not enough fresh air—any one of these and other insults to the body have been proved to be predecessors of a cold.

The ensuing cold is actually a health benefit, for it

acts as a safety valve. The periodic purification of colds can help keep down the debris that accumulates from poor health habits and thus prevent more serious disease.

The unpleasant symptoms of illness can often be cured by taking medicine, but this is not a real cure; it is merely the *suppression of symptoms*. The outward signs have been stopped, but the unhealthful conditions responsible for them remain unchanged. The signs have ended, but the malady lingers on.

The antidote that knocks out the "bug" also knocks out the body's efforts toward needed purification. The medicine which stops the coughing is really stopping the lungs from forcibly expelling harmful substances. (A study of 6,071 smokers showed that those who coughed developed lung cancer less often than the non-coughers.) The alcohol rub that reduces fever—that hinders one of the body's natural eliminative processes—may thereby prolong the illness.

Even the accompanying weakness and pain of eliminative illness serve a useful purpose. Creating discomfort is the body's way of saying: "Stop activity; stop eating; do nothing but rest. Give me the chance and I will straighten things out."

The animal heeds these signals by resting and fasting, taking nothing but water. Man would be wise to do the same. By resting and fasting for at least the first few days of illness, he relieves his system of energy-wasting chores. The body is then unhindered in carrying out its self-appointed task of expelling poisonous wastes.

By removing the underlying cause of sickness—toxic wastes, not germs—the body can restore itself to a state of health.

Am I implying that Pasteur's time-honored germ theory is false? Am I insinuating that the doctrine accepted by medicine for over one hundred years should be re-examined? Yes, I am.

Lest you think me presumptuous, I hasten to tell you that Pasteur's theory has been challenged by many. Numerous doctors, scientists, and other learned men have questioned the hypothesis that disease is caused by germs.

"In reality, it is not the bacteria themselves that produce the disease," said Dr. Royal Raymond Rife, developer of the microscope, "but we believe it is the chemical constituents of these microorganisms acting upon the imbalanced cell metabolism of the human body that in actuality produces the disease. We also believe that if the metabolism of the human body is perfectly balanced or poised, it is susceptible to *no* disease." [1]

Dr. Arnold Lorand says, in his book *Old Age Deferred*: ". . . that which we call disease is nought else but nature's attempt to attain health—a kind of defensive reaction against harmful substances. The disease proper has often already been present for some time; it already exists at the very instant in which the invading foe makes its entrance into the body." [2]

Pasteur's theory was disputed from the very start. Though hailed by most of the world as one of the greatest medical discoveries of all time, the germ theory expounded by Pasteur was immediately challenged by another scientist, Antoine Bechamp. Others have also disputed Pasteur's ideas down through the years, but to little avail, for Pasteur's opposition has garnered scant notice.

The germ theory of disease is still steadfast, and little wonder, for surface evidence tends to support the conten-

[1] *Prevention*, September, 1968.
[2] Dr. Arnold Lorand, *Old Age Deferred* (Philadelphia: F.A. Davis Co., 1926).

tion that the cause of infectious disease is bacteria. In infectious illness, bacteria are always present and active, and it is easy to conclude that they are the ailment's cause.

Further support to the germ theory seems to be given by the modern wonders achieved by public sanitation, antibiotics, and vaccination. Sanitation works by preventing germs from reaching human bodies. Antibiotics kill germs which have entered the body. Vaccination somehow helps the body to develop an immunity against certain germs. All this would appear to prove that germs are responsible for infectious illness. But stronger evidence contradicts the germ theory. Germs appear to be merely the triggering agents for a condition really brought about by faulty living habits. More logical than the germ theory is the *toxin-and-germ* theory. This theory says that infectious disease is caused by a *combination of accumulated toxins and the presence of germs.*

In order for infectious disease to start, two conditions must be present: (1) Through an accumulation of toxic wastes, the body must have become susceptible to certain germs, and (2) The appropriate germs must be present in the body in significant numbers. Both the explosive and the spark to set it off must be present. When either is missing, purification does not occur.

Proof of the toxin-and-germ theory's soundness abounds. It has been demonstrated in every epidemic. While some "catch" the disease, many others who are exposed avoid it. Those who avoid it are apparently the ones least in need of bodily purification. Some of those who have been exposed develop only a mild case of the disease. They seem to be the ones who have less need for cell purification.

Further proof of the toxin-and-germ theory is offered by the fact that all of us, at all times, harbor some disease germs within our bodies. Unemployed bacteria reside in all of us and become active only when the need arises. Dormant germs are living in the systems of people who are completely healthy.

The pneumonia germ is present in the mouths of 80 to 90% of the population. The tuberculosis germ has been carried by most of us at one time. The cold virus is generally present in everyone. If a germ is really the cause of a disease, how can one explain that many who carry the germ remain in good health?

During an epidemic, those who avoid the disease are said to have more resistance to it. This resistance is nothing more than the purer bodies that have been built by those who follow better living practices for one reason or another.

The power of proper living habits to resist disease is demonstrated by the informed minority of health-builders, some of whom are even immune to colds. Among those who do not practice healthful living habits deliberately, many do so unconsciously. A person may get eight hours' sleep nightly by preference or habit, his occupation may require muscular exertion, and he may happen to be the type who maintains a tranquil mind. This last factor alone could be enough to outweigh many deleterious living habits and make the person highly disease-resistant.

All of the foregoing is not meant to belittle antibiotics and vaccines, the germ-destroyers, nor to suggest their abolition. These germ-killing measures have brought extra years of life to many.

Even when their possible harmful side effects are taken into consideration, antibiotics are sometimes still the lesser evil and will be necessary as long as people continue to violate the laws of health. Similarly, vaccination against disease not caused by poor sanitation is still necessary for so long as Americans continue to follow unhealthful living practices.

An example of this is polio, the fundamental cause of which has been shown to be not the polio germ, but sugar. Sugar was proved to be the real culprit in 1948, even before the development of polio vaccine. A polio epidemic in the southeastern part of the country was halted by Dr. Benjamin Sandler, who through massive radio appeals convinced listeners to withhold from their diets the sugary foods that were polio's true cause. Further evidence against sugar as the real cause of polio is that the disease occurs most frequently and with greatest severity in those countries where sugar consumption is highest.

By creating an immunity against polio germs, vaccination has practically abolished polio, but the needle has not removed the underlying cause.

Better than vaccination against polio, which sometimes brings on bad side effects and even death, would be the removal from the diet of concentrated sugars responsible for polio. But well-meaning parents continue to let their children gorge on candy, soft drinks, pastries, and other highly sugared treats. For this reason, fighting the germs that trigger the disease is the lesser evil. Of course, this system still leaves the sugar-consuming child vulnerable to other sugar-caused diseases. The child saved from polio today is a potential heart-attack victim in later life.

The various germ-destroying measures don't remove the basic cause of disease: improper living habits. By failing to do so, they only put off the ultimate day of reckoning. It is better not to place your hope in germ exterminators which at best only postpone a day of atonement. It is far better to try to make yourself invincible to disease by frequent exercise, a tranquil mental attitude, proper diet, an occasional fast, and other such means of disease prevention.

All this has been a roundabout way to approach the last health and longevity influence, and a strange one it is. The final factor affecting good health and long life is *sickness.*

Be thankful for the minor infectious diseases that have come your way. They have helped to keep your system clear of debris. Their appearance on the scene is proof that they were needed. Minor illnesses prevent major illnesses. Minor illnesses can prolong life.

Even after you have embarked on your health and longevity program, your body may still at times seek to purify itself through eliminative illness. Regardless of your efforts toward right living, an occasional need for emergency bodily purification may still arise.

If minor eliminative illness occurs, it should cause you no misgivings. Instead, it should be looked upon as what it is, a purification process—a natural way of improving your health.

In his longevity studies, Dr. Raymond Pearl learned that not all of those who live long enjoy excellent health. Though few had undergone major surgery, a not inconsiderable proportion had been sickly. Superb health doesn't always accompany longevity. Apparently, those of the long-lived who had been sickly were so because they *needed* their ailments. Their minor maladies helped prevent more severe sicknesses.

If minor eliminative illness appears, you know what to do: Don't halt or hinder the natural symptoms by which your body seeks to restore health. If possible, help your body in its attempts at self-purification by resting and fasting for a few days.

Of course, if symptoms are severe enough to require the services of a doctor, you should obtain them. If and

when you need a doctor, try to find one familiar with
natural healing methods, who will cooperate with the
body's efforts at self-cure and who will interfere with
nature only if your symptoms become excessive.

Upon recovery, redouble your efforts to keep your body
purified and disease-resistant by practicing the secrets of
good health and long life.

SUMMARY

A bona fide and natural health and longevity factor is
minor eliminative illness, which can prevent major illness
and prolong life. If minor eliminative illness appears,
help your body in its attempts at self-purification by resting and fasting for a few days, instead of suppressing its
symptoms.

If symptoms are severe, see a doctor.

thirty-nine

The Mixed Bag

We return now to the point of this book: health and longevity are benefited by certain practices that copy the way of life established during more than one hundred thousand successive generations.

During mankind's first two million years on earth, his way of life remained essentially the same. Each man lived the same kind of life his father had, and as his ancestors had for thousands of generations before him. Even when man, a scant few thousand years ago, began to make discoveries that altered his living pattern, these changes did not, at first, greatly affect his basic way of life. It has been during only the twentieth century that the most pronounced and disruptive innovations have begun.

For the sake of health and longevity, we must return to a life style more like that of the past. Keeping modern civilization's many advantages, we need to return to some degree of "uncivilized" living. Such a life is simpler, pleasanter, and happier, as well as more healthful and of longer duration.

From the standpoint of its effects on health and longevity, civilization has been a mixture of both the good and the bad. Much can be entered on the credit side, for today countless conveniences ease the stress of living. Moreover, public sanitation has eliminated many former threats to health and life, and excellent medical service is readily available when needed.

But much of our progress is false. The same civilization that has blessed us with many advantages has also cursed us with the conveniences which keep us from exercising, with refined foods which short-change us of the nutrients we need, and with chemical pollution which sullies our bodies.

Former foes of health and long life are being subdued, but other cripplers and killers are taking their place. While conquering infant mortality and epidemic diseases, we of the twentieth century are losing the fight against a host of other disorders, ranging from tooth decay to heart disease and cancer.

Therefore, the enlightened few embrace whatever in civilization is beneficial to health and longevity, but forsake, as best they can, the detriments of the modern age. They accept the best, and reject the rest. Those natural-health factors which are missing from modern life, the wise few pursue on their own.

To make it easier for you to follow my system of health and longevity, the following is a condensed version of the Prohaska Plan, a summary of the nineteen main factors that have an influence on health and longevity:

1. Exercise—Walk, run, bicycle, or swim daily.

2. Mental Tranquility—Replace harmful emotions like worry, fear, anxiety, apprehension, and discouragement with beneficial emotions such as cheerfulness, hope, serenity, and satisfaction.

3. *Nutrition*—Avoid the devitalized or poisoned foods: white flour, white sugar, white rice, degerminated corn-meal, salt, cold-meat products, fish from inland waters, shellfish, coffee and tea. Eat little animal fat, more vegetable fat.

Eat some complete animal-protein food—meat, fish, milk, or eggs at every meal, and get at least half of your total food intake in raw form.

To keep your cells filled with every needed element, follow the Saturation Diet daily.

4. *Poison Avoidance*—Avoid ingesting chemical poisons as much as possible. The principal sources of poisons are insecticides applied to growing foods, chemicals added to food during processing, air pollution, medical drugs, cigarettes, and alcoholic beverages except when taken in strict moderation.

5. *Accident Avoidance*—Remember that most accidents represent a desire to hurt oneself, and convince yourself of the folly of this. Avoid potential accident situations, and discharge self-destructive tendencies harmlessly through expression and action.

6. *Sunshine*—Sunbathe outdoors frequently, spending part of the time in direct sunlight, the rest in the shade. Wear as little clothing as possible, and don't wear glasses outdoors. Don't overexpose in direct sunlight.

7. *Undereating*—Eat only when hungry, and stop eating while still a little hungry. Don't eat between meals.

8. *Fasting*—If you are in good health, fast for up to three days a few times a year. During minor illness, help nature cure you by fasting.

9. *Sleep*—Sleep at least eight hours each night, take a midday nap when possible, and go to bed early.

10. *Oxygen*—Spend as much time out-of-doors as pos-

sible. When indoors, ventilate well by opening the windows, and sleep with the windows open, or better still, sleep outdoors in a sleeping bag.

11. Overweight—To reduce weight cut down on carbohydrate and fat foods, and exercise.

12. Elimination—To help your skin aid the eliminative organs, induce heavy perspiration frequently through vigorous exercise or a sauna bath, but be certain to replace food elements lost from perspiring.

13. Aiding Blood Circulation—If possible, work in a seated position or while moving about on your feet. When standing or sitting for long periods, flush the leg veins by alternately raising heels and toes. Every hour or two, pause briefly, and prop your legs higher than your head. To flush your circulatory system, perform headstands, hang upside down while suspended by the legs, or hang by the hands from a horizontal bar, then bend over from the waist while standing with knees bent. The latter two exercises also stretch your spine.

14. Chewing—To chew your food thoroughly, take smaller mouthfuls, chew at a slower rate, and chew each mouthful longer.

15. Country Living—Country or small-town life is more conducive to health and longevity than city living. But if you are a city-dweller, you can gain many of the advantages of country living by following the Prohaska Plan.

16. Sickness—Minor eliminative illness can prevent major illness and prolong life. When you get a minor eliminative illness, help your body by resting and fasting for a few days. If the symptoms are severe, see a doctor.

17. Public Sanitation—Public sanitation, which prevents a great deal of disease and saves countless lives, is administered for you by the government. Support your government's sanitation laws.

18. *Medicine*—The medical profession stands ready to help you, if needed, but following the advice in these pages may eliminate most of the need for medical services.

19. *Heredity*—Your chances for longevity are enhanced if you come from long-lived ancestors, but a poor hereditary outlook can be overcome by diligently following the Prohaska Plan.

Most essential to your health and longevity are the first three factors listed in the foregoing paragraphs. The next ten are perhaps a little less influential, but are still extremely important. To pass over any of these principal health and longevity factors could be a grave mistake. Disease and premature death are probably the result of not just one, but a combination of causes in most cases.

The true causes of death are never traced. Death certificates list such causes as cancer or heart disease, but they never say lack of exercise, too much mental turmoil, a diet deficient in needed elements, on too little sunshine and fresh air.

Other factors which can also affect health and longevity, though probably to a lesser extent, are:

Level of income—People who have the advantages that come from a relatively high income are more often healthy and long-lived than those in lower-income groups. Among the probable reasons for this are that the well-to-do enjoy freedom from worries connected with limited finances and that they can afford the more expensive and more nourishing foods, instead of cheap, bulky carbohydrates.

Noise—The many noises produced by today's civilization create stresses detrimental to health and longevity.

Overcrowding—When the wild-animal population of a territory exceeds a certain ratio, a proportion of the apparently healthy animals sometimes die off, even though no discernible cause, such as food shortage, can be found for this. Some evidence seems to show that overcrowding among humans may foster similar consequences.

Certain groups would like you to think that many of the health pitfalls I have warned you against are nonexistent or exaggerated. Among these are various groups in the food industry, chemical interests, farmers' organizations, and other groups with financial interests at stake. These groups are well-organized, well-financed, and influential, and their puppets are skilled at creating persuasive publicity, often by the use of crafty techniques.

Sugar, an ad proclaims, is the food for your growing youngsters because it's an all-energy food. True, but it's also utterly devoid of the vitamins and minerals your children need.

Without insecticides, a magazine article claims, our farmers couldn't raise enough food to feed us all. If this were true, how did farmers get by before insecticides, and how do organic farmers manage to do so today?

Ordinary breakfast cereals, according to a nutritional authority quoted in a news item, provide a nourishing breakfast—if accompanied by milk and fruit juice. Of course, sawdust would also provide a nourishing breakfast if it were accompanied by milk and fruit juice, but the nourishment would come from the milk and the fruit juice.

Unlike those who contradict my statements, I will gain nothing financially, whether you follow my advice or not. My reward is helping you and your family become healthier and live longer. I share, with the late philosopher Bertrand Russell, an "unbearable pity for the suffering of mankind."

When you weigh the evidence, pro and con, please bear
in mind that the main interest of those who contradict my
theories is to sell you something, while my concern is with
the health and longevity of you and your loved ones.

forty

The Good Life

We search for the "causes" of tooth decay, cancer, heart trouble, and other scourges of humanity. We pin our hopes on ever-newer drugs, germ killers, and surgical techniques, but in the meantime, we violate all the established laws of natural living.

Think of it! While we spend billions searching for the answer to the riddle of disease, the simple, nonmedical, nonsurgical solution to many, if not most, of our health problems is right under our noses, ignored by nearly all and exploited by only an enlightened few.

True health cannot be found in the doctor's office, the hospital, or the drug store, although temporary relief sometimes can. You can achieve real health only through your own efforts. When you follow natural living habits, you provide your body with the conditions it needs to build its own health.

My new way of life can *renew* your life by giving you: better health, better spirits, and longer life.

Your improved health will be brought about mainly through actual internal physical alterations. Most of these beneficial changes will be wrought within you as the result of regular, vigorous physical activity. Exercise will create health-building internal transformations such as reduced arterial cholesterol, enlarged arteries, an increased number of capillaries, the creation of extra blood, reduced blood pressure, lower pulse rate, a larger, stronger heart, and cells that are saturated with oxygen.

Further beneficial changes will occur through the practice of good nutrition. With its emphasis on raw, unrefined, and complete foods, the Saturation Diet will charge your cells by supplying all the food elements your body needs for optimum health. An occasional fast will further alter you from within, by removing accumulated waste from your cells.

These magical bodily changes will transform you into a new person. In addition, your adoption of beneficial emotional habits will reduce the mental stress that can be a leading contributor to poor health. The influence of exercise and the other methods of working off tensions will help you alleviate the stresses you can't avoid.

Added to the various means of preventing or working off emotional stress are natural tranquilizing methods, such as exercise, which are further aids to mental serenity. Exercise somehow improves the spirits. The well exercised enjoy a happier state of mind, and a pleasurable feeling can swell to outright euphoria during actual exercise.

Additional mental serenity comes from regular and sufficient sleep, exposure to sunshine, and partaking of the natural and healthful tranquilizing foods, dolomite, brewer's yeast, and desiccated liver.

Taking advantage of these health and longevity secrets may add ten, twenty, thirty, or more healthful, happy years to your life.

Through exercise, mental tranquillity, regular intake of

Vitamin E, and the avoidance of white sugar, white flour, hydrogenated fat, salt, and cigarettes, you can all but eliminate the risk of heart disease, today's number one killer. By means of exercise, mental tranquillity, regular intake of Vitamin E, and the avoidance of chemical poisons, you can guard against cancer, the number two killer. Practice of all the secrets in these pages will help guard you against *all* killer diseases.

I am sometimes asked, "Wouldn't you rather get more fun out of life, even if it means you won't be so healthy or live so long?" The fun referred to is smoking, drinking, inactivity, and so forth. My reply goes something like this: "Getting more fun out of life is why I follow my way of living. It's fun to feel good. It's fun to feel full of pep. *Feeling* and *being* healthy is the most fun there is. It's no fun to be sick. It's no fun to drag around feeling half-alive. Feeling sick is the most miserable feeling there is."

It's true that cigarettes, liquor, and other stimulants provide a "lift," but this is only a temporary feeling, which you will pay for later. The enlightened few—through exercise, complete diet, achievement of mental tranquillity, periodic fasting, and the other health secrets—enjoy a constant feeling of elevation, and they get this stimulation with *benefit*, not harm, to their health and longevity.

Many never fully appreciate good health until they endure a serious illness. Only then do they really understand that when you have your health, you have everything. This thought was expressed in different words by a health-minded sage who prayed: "Dear Lord, give me good health, and I will take care of all the rest."

With its emphasis on vigorous exercise, radical diet, fasting, and other unorthodox living procedures, my system may be considered extremism by some, and they will be right. Extremism is what I am preaching. If you want moderate health and longevity, then practice moderation, but if you are after the extreme in health and longevity, practice extremism. Follow my advice in all its health-building, life-increasing, youth-restoring extremism. You will then be doing all you can to promote the utmost health and longevity.

You have now become one of the enlightened few. You now have the precious knowledge that can help you gain life's greatest blessings: health and longevity, plus that welcome bonus-benefit, better spirits. By practicing all these health and longevity secrets, you can grow healthier, happier, and in a sense, younger.

Your new-found know-how can help you reduce the need for medical services to a minimum, and perhaps enable you to avoid doctors, dentists, and hospitals, and the accompanying pain, inconvenience, and bills entirely. Like the enlightened elite, you may even gain freedom from headaches and colds.

The sooner you begin the good life, the sooner you will start to feel its benefits, and the sooner you will start to turn back the clock. The best time to start is right now. Today is the first day of the rest of your life. May this book help you to a long lifetime of health and happiness.

index

Accidents:
  as cause of death, 176–177
  chronic victims of, 178
  program for prevention of, 178–179, 241
  real cause of most, 177–178
Acerola berry, 93–94
Activity *See* Physical activity
Additives in food, 121–122
  how to avoid, 134–135
Air, need for fresh, 36–41
Air pollution, 124–127, 136
Alcohol, 116, 213
Alcoholism, 138, 139
  See also Drinking alcoholic beverages
Americans, 95–96
  medical expenses of, 7
  present diet of, 49, 63, 66
Amino acids, 86–87, 100, 109
Anger, importance of expressing, 172
Animal foods, daily need for, 105
Antibiotics, 235–236
Appendicitus, 4
Appendix, 228
Arteries, 194
Arthritis, 28
Aspirin, 122
Avidin, 100
Ayres, Dr. Stephen, 124

Back pain remedy, 24, 25
Bannister, Roger, 196
Baruch, Bernard, 209
Bechamp, Antoine, 233
Beri-beri, 69
Berkson, D. M., 222
Bierman, Dr. Howard R., 228
Big business, interests of, 145
Biotin, 100
Bishop, Dr. Louis F., 198
Blood pressure, 195
Bloodstream, 35–36, 216
Bogart, Larry, 144
Bone meal, 93, 105
Bragg, Paul, 2, 22, 148
Braithwaite, Dr. E. E., 157
Bread:
  white, 63, 66
  whole grain, 66, 68
Brewer's yeast, 88, 93, 105, 106, 174, 206
B vitamins, 100, 106, 140, 174, 206

Caffeine, 128
Calcium, 55–56, 93, 98, 107, 129, 206
Cancer, 228, 248
Cancer, possible causes of:
  chemical pollution, 116, 123
  emotional stress, 158

251

inadequate supply of oxygen, 37–38, 67, 185
lack of exercise, 184–185
smoking, 177
vitamin C deficiency, 55
vitamin E deficiency, 67–68
Cancer, skin, 32
Capillaries, 194–195
Carbohydrates, 52, 53, 106, 109, 211–213
Cereals, breakfast, 69–70, 244
"Certified raw milk," 99–100
Chapman, Dr. Carleton B., 199
Cheese, 102
Chemical poisoning, 115–129
how to avoid, 130–141
Chemical treatment of animals, 120–121
Chewing food properly, 108–111, 242
Chicken, 134
Chlorine, 128
Cholesterol, 80, 81–82, 100, 102, 194
Circulation of blood, 19–20, 242
exercises to aid, 22–25
Civilization, effect of, on health, 13–14, 239–240
Coffee, 127–128
Cohen, Phil, 3
Cold-meat products, 89–90, 91
Colds, causes of:
emotional upheaval, 157
excess table salt, 79
Colds, purification benefit of, 231–232
Condon, Richard, 148
Cooking food, 49, 54–57, 60
Cooper, Major Kenneth H., 190
Cooper sulphate, 128
Cornmeal, 69
Cow's milk, 100–101
need for, 97–98
pasteurization of, 98–99

Crying, importance of, 172
Cumler, Bill, 198–199
Cureton, Dr. Thomas K., 183–184, 198
Cyclamates, 118–119

Daily minium requirements, 104
Davis, Adele, 66–67, 98
DDT, 117–118
Death wish, 177
Defensive organs, 228
Dental health, 4
Desiccated liver, 93, 106, 174
Desserts, healthful, 92
DeVries, Herbert A., 209–210
Diet:
of Americans, 49, 53
of early man, 12
influence of, on health, 51–53
reducing, 212–214
Diseases, causes of, 230–238
Dodson, Bill, 196
Dolomite, 93, 105, 174
Drinking alcoholic beverages:
effect of, on health, 127
how to avoid danger of, 136–139
Drugs, 122–124, 128
Drury, Emma-Jane E., 70
Dubos, Dr. Rene, 46

Eggs, 85, 90, 100, 101–102
Elimination of wastes, 216–219, 231
Emotional tensions, ways of relieving, 171–175, 199–200
Emotions:
as cause of sickness, 156–161
how to avoid negative, 160, 162–170
Enzymes, 56–57, 98
Euphoria:
meaning of, vi
slow running as stimulant for, 192–193

Evolution of man, 12–14, 20–21, 30, 70–71, 94–95, 167–168
as argument for vegetarianism, 85
Exercise, 247
advice about, 188–193, 201–208
and heart disease, 198–199
most beneficial forms of, 190, 193, 240
for women and children, 208–209
Exercising for Physical Fitness (President's Council on Physical Fitness), 191, 192–193
Eyes, sunshine and, 28, 30

Fasting:
advice about, 151–155
reasons for, 147–150, 241
and reducing, 213–214
Fasting Can Save Your Life (Shelton), 149, 149n.
Fats, 52, 109–110, 211–213
See also Hydrogenation
Saturated fats
Unsaturated fats
Fever, 231
Fish, 90, 133–134
Fishbein, Morris, 55–56
Fletcher, Horace, 108
"Fletcherizing," 108–109
Flour, white, 63–64, 67
Fluorides, 129
Food and Nutrition Board of the National Research Council, 104
Food supplements, 95–96, 105–106
Fried foods, 82
Friendship, importance of, 173
Fruits, 57, 92, 105, 131

Gallup, Dr. George, studies of, 10, 15, 41, 42, 45, 85, 114, 148, 175, 180

Geriatrics magazine, 114
Germ theory of disease, 232–234
Giving, the need for, 174
Goals, lowering of, 164–166
Gout, 124–125, 127, 139, 154–155, 157–158
Grains, whole, 70–71
"Gravity break," 22
Guilt feelings, 166–169

Hanging upside down, 23–25
Happy, learning to be, 162–163
Happy People Rarely Get Cancer (Rodale), 158
Hardy, Dr. J.D., 29
Harris, Louis, 167
Headaches, a remedy for, 24
Headstands, 22–23
Health, recent upsurge of interest in, 9
"Health belt" of United States, 220
Health-food dealers, 69, 92, 102, 132
Healthful foods, 91–93
Heart, enlarged, 197–198
Heart disease, 198, 248
American epidemic of, 67, 182–184
emotional tension and, 158
excess salt as cause of, 79
excess sugar as cause of, 73
lack of exercise as cause of, 182, 183
Heredity, 15–18, 243
Herting, Dr. David C., 70
Heuper, Dr., 121
Hoffman, Bob, 209
Honey, 76
Hostility feelings, 168–169
Hunt, H. L., 2
Hunzans, 6–7, 11, 41, 42, 45, 46, 49–50, 66, 85, 114, 175, 180, 221
Hydrogenation, 79, 80–81

If You Must Smoke (Rodale), 174–175
Illness, minor, as aid to long life, 237–238, 242
Income level, as factor affecting health, 243
Inner biological rhythms, 46–47
Ivy, Dr. Andrew C., 127

Jackel, Dr. Merl M., 157
Juices, 60–62

Kelp, 93, 105, 206
Kidneys, effect of meat on, 88–89
Kinsey, Dr. Alfred, 168
Kleitman, Nathaniel, 43
Klumpp, Dr. Theodore G., 191
Knowledge boom, 142–144

Lacto-ovo-vegetarians, 85
Lacto-vegetarians, 85, 89
Lawrie, Macpherson, M.D., 72–73, 73n.
Lead, 124–127
Lear, John, 65
Let's Get Well (Davis), 66–67
Let's Live magazine, 69
Lewis, Larry, 2
Liebman, Rabbi Joshua, 164, 164n., 174
Life Extension Institute of Rutgers University, 42
Link, Henry C., Ph.D., 186–187, 187n.
Liver:
    effect of meat on, 88–89
    function and needs of, 140
Liver, desiccated. *See* Desiccated liver
Living habits and health, 12
Lobbyists, 145–146
Longevity:
    contributing factors of, vii, 5

and heredity, 15
and sunlight, 29
Longgood, William, 121
Lorand, Dr. Arnold, 233, 233n.
Lungs, 35

McCarrison, Sir Robert, 6–7, 50–51, 53, 184
Macfadden, Bernarr, 16–17, 22, 45, 148
McGrady, Pat, 123–124
MacMitchell, Les, 196
McVay, Dr. Jay R., Jr., 228
Mann, Dr., 88–89
Maple sugar, 77
Mason, Harry, 2–3
Mayer, Jean, Ph.D., 185
Meares, Ainslie, M.D., 166–167, 167n.
Meat, 88–89, 105
Meat-eating, 84–89
Medical profession, 10, 226–227, 229
Medicines, 116, 122, 139, 232, 243
Mental origin of ailments, 156–161
Mental tensions, how to discharge, 171–175
Mental tranquility, 175, 240
Milk, 85, 90, 100–101, 105 *See also* Cow's milk
Milk, raw, 98–100
Millet, Dr., 37
Minerals, 52, 55–56, 74, 96, 98, 107, 206
Mitchell and Hamilton, 88
Molasses, blackstrap, 76

Nagorny, Professor A., 209
Nap-taking, 44–45
Narcotics, 129
Natural Food and Farming, 132, 133
Natural foods, 12, 74, 78

Nature Hits Back (Macpherson), 72–73, 73n.

Nebraska, elderly residents of, 11, 220–221

Newburgh and Johnston, 88

Noise, as detriment to health, 243

No Miracles Among Friends (Ogilvie), 158, 158n.

Nuclear power, 144

Nurmi, Paavo, 196

Nutrition, 12–13, 48–53, 107, 241

Nutritionists, 12

Nuts and peanuts, 59, 82, 88, 105

Obesity, causes of, 211–215, 242

Ogilvie, Sir Heneage, 158, 158n.

Oils:
    hydrogenation of, 79, 80–81
    refined, 66, 80
    unhydrogenated, 69, 106

Old age, studies of, 10–11

Old Age Deferred (Lorand), 233, 233n.

Organic foods, 132–134

Organic Gardening magazine, 132, 133

Osteomalacia, 27

Ott, Dr. John, 28–29

Outdoor living, 40–41

Overcrowding, as detriment to health, 244

Overweight. *See* Obesity

Oxygen, 35–36, 241–242

Oxygen deprivation, as cause of cancer, 37–38

Pasteur's germ theory, 232–234

Patterson, Clair C., 125

Peace of Mind (Liebman), 164, 164n.

Pearl, Dr. Raymond, 5, 11, 15, 137–138, 139, 195, 196, 237

Pederson, P.O., 74

Perspiration, 217–218

Pesticide poisoning, how to avoid, 130–132, 152–153

Pesticide sprays, 120

Phenols, 123–124

Physical activity:
    effects of, on body, 194–200
    as most important health and longevity factor, 180–187
    need for, by elderly, 209–210
    present lack of, 181–182
    for relief of emotional stress, 172–173, 186, 199–200
    studies of, 182–183

Plant foods needed daily, 105

Pleasures of Fasting, The (Condon), 148

Poisons:
    cumulative effect of, on body, 117–118
    how to avoid, 130–141, 241
    See also Chemical poisoning

Poisons in Your Food, The (Longgood), 121

Polio, 236

Prevention magazine, 69, 132, 191, 191n.

Price, Dr. Weston, 11, 41, 74, 184, 221

Prohaska, Aline, 4

Prohaska family, 3–4, 6

Proteins, 52, 84–90, 106, 109

Provoker, The, 186

Psychosomatic causes of ailments, 156–161

Pulse rate, 5, 195–197

Purification of cells, 216

Raw foods, 57–62

Refining foods, 49, 51, 63–71, 72, 73

Relief Without Drugs (Meares), 166–167, 167n.

Rice, whole brown, 69

Rickets, 27–28
Rife, Dr. Royal Raymond, 233
Rodale, J. I., 158, 174–175
Rosenbaum, Dr. Jean, 177
Running, advice about, 201–202
Rural life, as aid to better health, 221–223, 242
Russell, Bertrand, 244
Russian centenarians, studies of, 11, 114

Salt:
  in baby food, 80
  effect of, on diet, 79–80
  loss of, during exercise, 205
  substitutes for, 80
Sandler, Dr. Benjamin, 236
Sanitation, public, 224–225, 240, 242–243
Saturated fats, 80–82
Saturation Diet, 104–107
Sauna baths, 218
Schaller, George, 94
Schweigart, Dr. H.A., 37
Seeds, edible, 59, 88, 105, 131–132
Selye, Dr. Hans, 199–200
Sex, as cause of guilt feelings, 167–168
Shaw, George Bernard, 22, 85
Shellfish, 90
Shelton, Dr., 149
Sherman, Dr. Henry C., 104
Shubik, Dr. Philippe, 116
Shute brothers, 67
Side Effects of Drugs, 123
Sinclair, Upton, 85
Sitting during work, 19, 21
Skin:
  effect of sunshine on, 27
  as eliminative organ, 217–219
Slack, Dr. Geoffrey L., 75
Sleep, 241
  best surface for, 45

best time for retiring, 45–46
  need for eight hours per night, 42–44
Smoking cigarettes, 115–116, 117, 127, 136, 232
Social Security Agency's study of centenarians, 11, 41
Sofka, Michael, 17–18
Solar house, 33
Soy protein, 87
Spies, Dr. Tom, 174
Spinal column, 23
Stagg, Amos Alonzo, 209
Standing, effect of, on health, 19–21, 25
Stilbestrol, 121
Strength and Health magazine, 209
Strontium, 152, 153
Studies of Long-lived people, 10–12
Sugar:
  brown, 77
  as cause of polio, 236
  raw, 77
  substitutes for, 76–78
  white, 63–65, 72–73, 244
Sunbathing in winter, 32–33
Sunshine, 106, 241
  health-giving qualities of, 26–31
  overexposure in, 31–32
Supplement potencies, 107
Surgery, avoidance of, 227–228
Sweeteners, unharmful, 76–78

Talking problems out, 173
Tea, 127–128
Technocrats, 144
Teeth, brushing of, 75
Terry, Surgeon-General, 117
Thiamine, 174–175
Thoughts, learning to control one's 160, 162–164

Thymus gland, 228
Tobe, John, 138, 186
Today's Health, 165
Tonsils, 227–228
Tooth decay, 4, 28
    food processing as cause of,
    73–76
Toxin-and-germ theory of di-
    seases, 234–235
Tranquilizers:
    artificial, 122, 123
    exercise as, 191–193
    natural, 174–175
    sunshine as, 27
Tuberculosis, 37

Ulcers, 159
Undereating, benefits of, 112–
    114, 241
United States Government:
    Congress, address of, 146
    President, address of, 146
    and protection against chemi-
    cal poisons, 144–146
Unsaturated fat, 80, 82, 106

Vaccines, 235–236
Vegetables, 58–59, 61, 105, 131
Vegetarianism, 84–89
Ventilation, 38–39

Vitamin A, 106
Vitamin B. *See* B vitamins
Vitamin C, 55, 61, 94–95, 98,
    105, 106, 140, 205–206
    importance of, during a fast,
    153
Vitamin D, 27–28, 30, 106
Vitamin E, 66–68, 69, 70, 106,
    107, 140, 182, 248
Vitamin supplements, 9
Vitamins, 52, 55, 98, 104, 106

Walking, importance of, 188–
    189
Warburg, Dr. Otto, 37
Water, drinking, 139, 151
    poisons in, 128–129
Weger, George S., M.D., 149,
    149n.
Wheat, 71
Wheat germ, 71, 88
Wheat residue, nutrients in, 65–
    66
White, Dr. Paul Dudley, 67
Whole-grain products, 68–69,
    105
Winklestein, Dr. Warren, 124
Women's need for exercise, 208

Yakovlev, N.N., 206
Yudkin, Dr. John, 73